UNDER THE GUN

UNDER THE GUN

An ER Doctor's Cure
for America's Gun Epidemic

Cedric Dark, MD, MPH
with Seema Yasmin, MB BChir

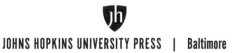

JOHNS HOPKINS UNIVERSITY PRESS | Baltimore

Johns Hopkins University Press
2715 North Charles Street
Baltimore, Maryland 21218
www.press.jhu.edu

Library of Congress Cataloging-in-Publication Data is available.

A catalog record for this book is available from the British Library.

ISBN 978-1-4214-4911-1 (hardcover)
ISBN 978-1-4214-4912-8 (ebook)

Special discounts are available for bulk purchases of this book. For more information, please contact Special Sales at specialsales@jh.edu.

For

Jan, Billy, Hamp, Chris
Robbie and Renita

In Memoriam

Robert Louis Scales III

In Memoriam

Dr. Tamara O'Neal

Knowledge which is unable to support action is not genuine—and how unsure is activity without understanding.

RUDOLF VIRCHOW

CONTENTS

CONTENTS

UNDER THE GUN

Prologue

In 2020, while the COVID-19 pandemic raged, altering the course of our collective lives, a steadily growing epidemic continued to burn its path across the United States at an ever-quickening pace. Gun violence—a term too easily misunderstood—stole the lives of 45,222 Americans that fateful year, which was the worst year on record for gun deaths to that point, according to data from the Centers for Disease Control and Prevention.

The path leading to each one of these deaths is layered and complex. Each American killed by a bullet, each family grieving their loved one, deserves their own book. I never once thought that I would be one to write such a story. I'm a gun-owning emergency physician, a father, and the cousin of a man who was shot to death. I still felt that there were many people more qualified to write this book: researchers, community organizers, survivors.

If it wasn't for the National Rifle Association declaring that physicians, like me, should "stay in their lane" and keep quiet about the toll of this plague on our communities, I wouldn't have written this book. Gun violence consumes my life. I see victims of gun violence from family tragedies—children, adolescents, and adults—almost every day. I am well within my rights to talk about this crisis. And I am not a novice to this topic.

Although gun violence prevention didn't become a years-long passion for me until the NRA sent that foolish tweet, I had already spent years examining how we can save lives and how we can use evidence-based policies to make this country safer before I joined the chorus of health care workers across America to collectively declare that #ThisIsOurLane.

Addressing violence and death is the duty of anyone who has ever had to mend the wounds of a gunshot victim, to attempt heroic measures in the trauma bay, to meticulously care for the injured in the intensive care unit, or admit defeat in front of their loved ones. I have found no worse feeling than having to tell a mother or a father that their child has been killed by a bullet. The visceral screams of those parents will haunt me forever.

My coauthor, Dr. Seema Yasmin, nudged me to retrace my own steps in this transformation, going back to my childhood to uncover a memory I had buried, a story that plunged me into this fight before I even took my first steps toward becoming a healer. She encouraged me to transform my righteous indignation about the disease of violence that annually brings over 600 gunshot victims into my own emergency department into a constructive storytelling platform to change the narrative around this politically charged topic. In addition to working as an emergency room doctor, I am trained in public health, the path I undertook to help me understand the root causes of illness. By the time a person becomes a patient in my ER, we have already failed them. My public health training enables me to ask, What led them to fall sick in the first place and how do we protect their health once they leave the hospital?

In thinking this way, I have been heavily influenced by the writing of the nineteenth-century German physician Rudolf Virchow, who said: "Medicine is a social science and politics is nothing else but medicine on a large scale. Medicine as a social science, as the science of human beings, has the obligation to point out problems and to attempt their theoretical solution; the politician, the practical anthropologist, must find the means for their actual solution."[1]

Our politicians, however, refuse to solve the problem of gun violence. Stuck between those who feel that the Second Amendment was declared by God Himself and others who want to ban certain types of firearms altogether, we cannot seem to speak reasonably to our better selves. So the task falls on the medical profession to right these wrongs. Virchow foresaw this. "If medicine is to fulfill her great task, then she must enter the political and social life."[2]

It may sound controversial, especially to some of my fellow physicians, but it's not just me calling us to step away from the trauma bay and into political discourse to address our patients' social determinants of health; it was Virchow.

We have practiced and perfected evidence-based medicine for decades. We should similarly practice evidence-based health policy. As it pertains to guns, some of the evidence for action already exists. While the NRA vainly attempts to discredit the work of our colleagues who have spent their lives and careers grappling with this phenomenon, we know how to analyze the data for ourselves. We know what to do to save the lives of our patients, and by extension, our communities.

We don't have to wait. We simply must realize that addressing gun violence is within our lane as health care workers. If you believe, as I do, that faith without works is dead, then shouldn't action trump thoughts and prayers?

I pray that my story will make you take action. I lean on mentors, on teachers, on colleagues, on friends, and even on neighbors to tell the only story I know how to tell—one of a physician and a policy-wonk-turned-advocate working to end gun violence. My story has evolved to learn the difficult truth that statistics lose out to narrative. And so to get the next American worshipper, school kid, festivalgoer, parade watcher, or bank customer out from under the gun, I'm writing this story in the hope that you will realize that this is your lane too.

CHAPTER ONE

Trauma

The phone rang too early that summer morning. My cousin Jan wasn't the kind of person to get out of bed, walk across her bedroom, and pick up the phone—not when the room was still dark and she had a job interview in a few hours. But something didn't feel right. The ring of the phone was too shrill, and the room suddenly felt cold. *Something* was wrong; she knew it.

"Jan," her father said through the phone. "Your brother is dead. Someone shot Robbie." Every word my Uncle Robert whispered after that—every word about the son to whom he had gifted his own name—sounded muffled to Jan, as if she was listening to her father speak through the din of a firing squad.

Robbie was young and handsome, a charming and dutiful son. He was six feet tall, an army reservist with a physically intimidating stature at over 220 pounds. Tuesday night, after wrapping up work at the local newspaper, the *Winston-Salem Journal*, Robbie had gone for a beer at a bar on the east side of the small North Carolina town. He was taking a sip of beer in that town built on tobacco when the phone rang. If only it had been a friend asking if they could join him at the bar. Instead, whatever was said on the other end of that phone made Robbie jump out of his seat and run to his car.

Robbie drove across town to his girlfriend's apartment. But his girlfriend wasn't alone. Another man was in her apartment causing a scene.

Anticipating a conflict, Robbie had brought his gun.

According to my mother, my cousin Robbie had always had an issue with his temper. It began with words, escalating to shouting, all attempting to lay claim to the woman in whose apartment the two men argued. Inside the cramped apartment, the man reached for Robbie's pistol. As the two men scuffled, each fighting to wrap his fingers around the narrow grip of the gun, the pistol was turned until the barrel of Robbie's own firearm was pointed straight at him. A single shot was fired into his belly. Just like that, my cousin was dead.

Decades have elapsed. Jan's face is now weathered with fine lines. Gray strands streak through her once jet-black hair. I pressed her and her brother Billy to talk about that hot summer morning that unfolded some 25 years ago. They had never spoken to me about it before.

"What else did your dad say? Why did he call you in the morning? Why didn't he call you that night? Can you remember how you felt?"

Numb, says Jan. She was numb. Enveloped in grief and confusion, the details of that day, of that month, of Robbie's burial, are cloaked in a walled-off sadness that is difficult to penetrate.

My Uncle Robert, Jan and Robbie's father, also never spoke of the day Robbie was killed. In fact, he never spoke of his son to me ever again.

Some people try to silence trauma. Some run from it, gas pedal to the ground, fleeing from one town to the next or one coast to another, putting thousands of miles between them and the thing pushing them into a purple grief. Some people mute the pain and dial down the volume—sometimes with alcohol, drugs, or other distractions—as months, years, and anniversaries pass. For others, trauma is like a train wreck; it hooks our gaze. We can't stop examining events from one angle and then another, like movie directors shooting a scene. We traipse through the rubble, lifting and interrogating every piercing shard, turning events over in our mind and parsing moments of pain as if they are debris. We long to fix what has been shattered.

Long before I was an emergency physician and a medical educator with an alphabet soup of letters after my name, I was a nerdy, four-eyed teenager whose cousin was shot dead. I didn't know much about trauma then. I knew about SATs and MCATs, the Baltimore Orioles and the Washington Bullets, the latter a team whose moniker would change in the mid-1990s so the flurry of gun violence penetrating the community where I lived wouldn't be glorified in the nickname of a sports franchise.

I didn't grow up in North Carolina, where most of my family lived. My parents, who both grew up in the small city of Winston-Salem, had long ago moved out to stake a life of their own, settling in the relative peace of Maryland's Prince George's County—known as the richest predominantly Black county in the nation by the time I was born. I spent my weekdays at a magnet school for techies and my weekends either at my house or a friend's house, writing short stories, playing video games, and eating ramen noodles. I dreamt of the years ahead of me and prepared for a life filled with science, microscopes, and medicines—thinking I would one day cure cancer, the disease that had taken one of my favorite aunts from me.

Robbie's death ruptured the peace. It ricocheted through my teenaged mind, reverberated through my growing body like an alarm clock. Subconsciously—although it's sometimes hard to trace our decisions to their exact roots—I think my cousin's death launched me into a career of confronting trauma, of looking it right in the eyes. I wasn't particularly close to Robbie—he lived two states away—but Robbie was my blood. I didn't attend the funeral. I hate funerals. And I hate death. Maybe that's why I joined a profession and a specialty that constantly battles against mortality.

When my mother returned from the funeral, she told me about the white gloves Robbie was wearing in his casket. The gloves were there to cover up the wounds on his hands that would never have the chance to heal, she said. I have never stopped thinking about that and imagining those never-healing wounds in my mind's eye. As a physician, I have seen countless similar injuries.

After high school, I left the Maryland suburbs for college in Georgia and then went to New York City for medical school and public health training. I carried with me that vicarious memory of Robbie lying in his casket and my family's silent, impenetrable grief.

Then, another crisis, another trauma introduced me to the emergency room soon after I began medical school. One morning from my perch on the roof of New York University's Rubin Hall on East 30th Street in Manhattan, I watched the Twin Towers burn in an act of violence so severe that it prompted a war. That day, September 11, 2001, I chose to dedicate my life to emergency medicine so I could learn how to piece together broken things: memories, bones, lives. Life is filled with crisis, I thought. I wanted to be useful in that moment when everything else was falling apart.

When I was fully qualified, after completing a four-year residency training program in emergency medicine and another three years practicing independently at Saint Agnes Hospital in West Baltimore, I moved to Houston to work as an attending emergency physician at the city's top trauma center. Our hospital is ranked as one of the best in the nation when it comes to saving the lives of trauma victims. Day and night, I grapple with death, grief, and often guns. I see people who remind me of my cousin Robbie every day; other people's cousins, brothers and sisters, sons and daughters, grandchildren writhing in the trauma bay, their breath slipping away beneath my gloved fingertips. On average, fourteen gunshot victims are wheeled into my hospital each week. Every month, six people die from a bullet wound in my emergency department. In 2020, when all the numbers were tallied across every community in the United States, the total was over 45,222 Americans who died from a bullet that year.[1] Not included in such tallies are the tens of thousands of Americans who suffer gun injuries and whose lives are robbed of peace, freedom, health, and joy.[2] Provisional estimates from the Centers for Disease Control and Prevention indicate that the number of deaths continues to climb.[3]

I am sure that you have heard these numbers before. Americans own close to 400 million guns, more than enough for every single man, woman, and child in the country.[4] In India, which ranks second on the global list of gun ownership, there is one gun for every twenty people. To me, it makes more sense to compare American civilians to global militaries. Tallying all the firearms in the hands of American civilians, our guns outnumber the guns in the possession of every military of every other country across the globe. Because American citizens own more firearms than the rest of the world's professional militaries combined, it is no surprise that over 120,000 of us are wounded or killed by firearms each year.

But this is not a book about statistics; this is a book about *stories*. Starting with my own and including the stories of my patients and my colleagues who have become too intimately acquainted with gun violence, this book is an investigation of how we got into this mess and how we can get out.

While some numbers will help us make sense of what we're up against, you can find the statistical reports elsewhere. I want to go beyond the datasets, death certificates, and medical reports, into the lives of ordinary Americans whose lives have been forever changed by gun violence and the doctors, like me, who come face-to-face with violence every day. In my work as a physician-advocate, I have learned that numbers might grab someone's attention, but it is stories that stick and provide hope for change.

We all make assumptions, whether we think we know the politics and personalities of gun owners or the people who want to see guns banned. This book interrogates those misconceptions. Beginning with me.

***

I'm firmly in my 40s now. I'm a Black man living in Texas, a father, a husband, a doctor—and I own guns. I even enjoy shooting guns. I respect them as weapons for sport, for hunting, and as a means of self-protection. This book isn't a treatise against guns or the Americans who enjoy them. This is the story of my life's work at the coalface of gun violence in America. It's the origin story of our collective denial about the endemic violence we are facing. It's a book that seeks to answer these questions: If we now lose more Americans to gun violence than car crashes each year, how can we remedy this tragedy? How have so many of us become numb to the loss of our fellow Americans? How can we maintain our individual right to own guns and still protect the lives of men, women, and children who die from a bullet each day?

Physicians are trained to pay close attention to the sick or injured person in front of them, to ask the right questions about their life and listen deeply to their pain. We're taught to make careful and nonjudgmental assessments of our patient's circumstances and environment. We piece together everything we see, smell, and hear, reading body language and facial tics, to make a diagnosis and write a prescription to treat the problem.

This book contains my careful observations and diagnoses of America's unique gun violence problem—an epidemic that singles America out from every other nation in the world. Based on two decades of work in emergency departments—including my life experiences during my teenage years when my cousin's gun was turned against him and my life as a father of a young Black boy in Texas—this is my invitation for you to enter the emergency department, to visit my neighborhood, to see what I see. Along the way, I will tell the stories of other physicians—some alive, some who died from bullet wounds—to understand how we can arrive at solutions to this problem.

These chapters offer a set of policy prescriptions, ideas for a healthier and safer way for America to coexist with firearms. Starting with a different way of framing the debate about gun violence—as a public health problem that can be navigated with the same tools used to stop the spread of infectious disease—this book offers evidence-based approaches that could help Americans regain the two-and-a-half years of life expectancy we lose to gun violence.[5]

I've already lived longer than my cousin Robbie. I want my son to have that same chance. I want him to enjoy the life expectancy of men living in Japan, Switzerland, and Australia, not to die a decade sooner, as is the life expectancy of a Black man in America. I want to drive my son to baseball practice at Emancipation Park without suffering the fate of Carmelo Duncan, the one-year-old boy who was killed by a stray bullet while in the back seat of his father's car as they drove through Washington, DC, in December 2020.

I want my son to focus on the next batted baseball on spring Saturday mornings instead of stumbling over a spent brass shell casing lying on the field from the previous night's violence. It amazes me how often I come across spent shells when on casual weekend walks in my neighborhood and how close danger comes to my own home. Come Monday morning, I will likely have seen another Carmelo or a Robbie in my emergency department. My hope is that by sharing their stories and offering these policy prescriptions, this book can help us create a safer, better future for all our children.

CHAPTER TWO

Contagion

Gun violence, a daily occurrence in communities across the United States, remains relatively uncommon in other parts of the world. If doctors in a country where gun violence is rare were to note an uptick in people who were shot, they might alert authorities to find out why a surge in cases was occurring. Physicians are often the first to notice when something strange is brewing in a community.

Dr. Li Wenliang, a Chinese doctor, noticed something strange occurring at his clinic in December 2019. As he dripped medicine into eyes and peered into pupils, Li's patients coughed and spluttered; he had to step back as they wiped their damp foreheads. His patients felt it was just the flu or maybe a really bad cold, but to Li, it didn't look or sound like a regular chest infection. He had flashbacks to the SARS epidemic of his teenage years.

When Li was just a teen in 2002, a new and mysterious illness swept across China, eventually zigzagging its way across oceans to infect people in India, Australia, and more than two dozen countries around the globe. Feverish patients coughed and gasped for air as the pathogen, a coronavirus that had spread from animals to humans, caused an outbreak of severe acute respiratory syndrome, or SARS. It infected the lungs of more than 8,000 people and killed almost 800.

Seventeen years later and a thousand miles away from the hot zone that sparked the 2002 epidemic, Li was a practicing physician specializing in the treatment of eye disease in a hospital in Wuhan, China. He was 34 years old; his wife was expecting their second child.

Li noticed his patient's lungs were filling with fluid, their blood vessels widening and jamming with sticky blood. Scans of their chests showed what looked like ground glass, a haze patching over the normally clear spaces inside their lungs.

Li rang the alarm, but officials in Wuhan did not heed his warning. "This could be the second coming of SARS," Li said in an online group chat of his medical school classmates. Li's friends listened when he said his patients were being sent home, where they were infecting their children, parents, and grandparents. Relatives of his patients wound up trapped in isolation in the intensive care unit on ventilators, breathing machines that artificially pump high concentrations of oxygen into the lungs. Although they listened on WeChat, the Chinese social media giant, there wasn't much Li's former medical school classmates could do.

On December 30th, Li sent a highly personal update: "Quarantined in the emergency department."[1] But infection wasn't his only concern. Local authorities were closing in on him. While Li was trying to sound the alarm on a new infectious disease, police accused him of spreading rumors and the government ordered his arrest. By then the virus was expanding its reach, sickening thousands of people across Wuhan. A few weeks after he first noticed the signs of a new contagion, Li contracted the virus from one of his patients. Doctors around the world began gathering personal protective equipment. The international community heeded Li's hospital-bed warnings and watched in horror as he grew sicker.

"SARS might come back. We needed to be ready for it mentally. Take protective measures," Li told the *New York Times* in January 2020 through an oxygen mask as he lay profusely perspiring in the hospital, infected with the virus he was trying to stop.[2]

As death and disease shuttered borders and brought global economies to a halt, scientists ramped up the search for a solution that could end the contagion. On January 11, 2020, just days after Li had first warned about the return of SARS, Chinese scientists decoded the genetic blueprint of the novel virus: it was indeed another coronavirus, a close relation to the original SARS virus. Li had been the harbinger of the new global health crisis.

Without Li's warnings rippling around the world—without the new virus scooped from the blood of the dead, its genetic code unraveled and shared freely with scientists around the world—the hunt for a vaccine could have taken a decade or more, the usual time it takes for vaccine development. Instead, multiple vaccines were being injected into arms in December 2020, just twelve months after Li sounded the alarm.

But before vaccines could be developed, on February 7, 2020, as the new coronavirus continued its journey across China and throughout the world, Li, straight black hair askew and a ragged mustache forming on his unshaven youthful face, took his last breath and died from COVID-19.

***

What does COVID-19 have to do with guns? In my opinion, America's gun violence crisis has a lot in common with epidemics of infectious disease. Had Li's early warnings been taken seriously by Wuhan authorities, had they helped Li investigate the strange symptoms and implemented early quarantines instead of silencing him, COVID-19 might have been contained to Wuhan or its surrounding areas in central China's Hubei province. Instead, the virus spread relentlessly across borders, killing millions of people across the planet. What could have been controlled as an isolated cluster of a novel disease spiraled out of control and became a global pandemic.

"If the officials had disclosed information about the epidemic earlier," Li told reporters days before his death, "I think it would have been a lot better. There should be more openness and transparency."

Just as Li attempted to warn the world of an imminent threat, physicians in the United States have been trying to ring the alarm about America's escalating gun violence for decades. Some call it an epidemic; others say that deaths from guns are so steeped into the fabric of America that we cannot use that term. I suggest that, rather, gun violence is endemic to America— a predictable disease that occurs regularly across the country at a baseline rate. Either way, we are past the point of containing this crisis to a small cluster; it is already a widespread phenomenon. Lessons learned from fighting outbreaks of infectious disease can be applied to America's gun crisis. A public health approach to violence should provide a way out of this national catastrophe, the same approach we have previously used with infectious diseases such as HIV and traumatic diseases such as motor vehicle collisions.

As an emergency physician, I can only heal one person at a time. I trained for four years after completing medical school to treat the single patient in front of me using all the modern medical technology at my disposal. If that patient were a child with measles, I would treat the symptoms of that illness—breathlessness, fever, rash, confusion, seizures—to make sure the child lived to see their next birthday.

Public health doctors take a different approach. Instead of the single-patient strategy, public health professionals take care of entire populations: communities, states, countries, and, as we saw during the COVID-19 pandemic, the entire world. Instead of treating the child struggling to breathe because of the measles virus, public health doctors think about ways to prevent millions of children from contracting measles in the first place.

Public health employs this big-picture approach. It operates in the background and rarely gains the praise it deserves. If it were not for the coronavirus pandemic, I imagine most Americans wouldn't give public health a second thought.

Meanwhile, Americans often imagine their physicians as lifesavers, heroic caregivers, and skillful surgeons who make snap decisions and perform dramatic and bloody procedures. While I might see one child with a severe case of measles and use medicines or perhaps plastic breathing tubes to treat the child's breathlessness and save that child's life, public health doctors toil away invisibly. Mass vaccination campaigns, helmed by public health professionals, have stopped measles from killing more than 21 million children in just the first two decades of the twenty-first century.[3]

The attacks we have witnessed against public health during the COVID-19 pandemic are akin to threatening the fire department with closure because the town hasn't seen a fire in months. "There have been no fires because we've been preventing fires from ever starting!" you can imagine a fire fighter saying. "We install smoke detectors; we teach kids not to play with matches." That's how public health works. Underfunded and easily misunderstood, its role is downplayed because so much of public health is about preventing people from winding up as patients in the first place. Public health is not like its sexier cousins, emergency medicine and trauma surgery, which have featured in scores of TV shows casting handsome actors such as Alan Alda, George Clooney, or Patrick Dempsey. As a Black kid growing up in the 1990s, I looked up to Eriq La Salle's character, Peter Benton, a surgeon with an epic hospital-hallway fist punch.

***

I had been drawn to emergency medicine ever since my first weeks in medical school in New York City. It wasn't long after my arrival in New York in August 2001 that I witnessed firsthand the incomprehensible devastation of the 9/11 terrorist attacks. I vividly remember that Tuesday morning. The sky was a crystal-clear blue, punctuated only by the smoke rising from the southern tip of Manhattan. My fellow first-year medical students and I swiftly sprang into action, rushing to Bellevue Hospital in the hope of being helpful on that fateful day. Of course, we were of little actual use.

Years later, during the massive Northeast Blackout of 2003, during a series of hot, sweaty summer nights, I was lured back to the chaos of emergency medicine. Doctors and nurses cared for New Yorkers in the jammed hallways of New York University's dimly lit and overheated emergency room. Ever since then, I have wanted to help the breathless, bleeding, confused patient in front of me, the person whose existence was suddenly ripped apart by something dire and unexpected. As I rotated through Bellevue and learned from legends such as

Dr. Lewis R. Goldfrank, I began to understand that the population approach of public health was just as important as the work I did in the emergency setting. The actions of public health doctors could impact what I would see—and not see—in my emergency department.

In medical school, we only spent a few short weeks learning the basics of public health, including the foundation of the discipline: epidemiology. The word epidemiology breaks down like this: *epi* is Greek for *upon, dem* means for *the people*, and *ology* refers to *the study* of something. *Epidemiology*, therefore, is the study of the trends and patterns of all the things that can afflict people. The public health doctor eyeing a patient with measles in the emergency room sees not only the child; she sees the teacher, siblings, grandparents, and friends who were close to the child; she sees the crowded bedroom the child shares with brothers and sisters; she sees the mother who struggled to take time off work to bring the child to the emergency department but was unable to take the time off to get routine vaccinations. She traces all the events that led to that child's emergency department visit, and she uses those same skills to think about patients who were injured at work or shot outside their homes. She connects the dots between a person's well-being or illness and their environment, and instead of seeing the person in isolation, she thinks of all the other people that person is connected to. Infectious diseases such as measles, COVID-19, and malaria as well as injuries such as motor vehicle crashes, falls, and gunshots can all be approached with the same meticulous public health methodology.

In her former role, my colleague and coauthor Dr. Seema Yasmin was an epidemic intelligence service officer at the Centers for Disease Control and Prevention (CDC), where epidemiologists study suicide trends, workplace injuries, trends in car traffic accidents, the use and effects of dietary supplements, patterns of violence, and much more.

Epidemiologists even study guns, as do physicians, health services researchers, and many scientists across a broad array of disciplines. But studying gun violence has become a touchy subject, partly because of emergency physicians.

"Firearms are fascinating pieces of equipment. I enjoy the sport of shooting, although I rarely shoot anymore," Dr. Arthur Kellermann told *Emory Magazine* in 1995.[4] "My dad taught me how to shoot when I was eleven or twelve years old," he said, as he described growing up around guns in a small town in rural eastern Tennessee. As a young man in the 1980s, Kellermann's love for firearms conflicted with his intellectual curiosity. He scratched his head, wondering how the guns he enjoyed for recreational fun led so many people to wind up as patients in his emergency department and in the county coroner's office.

"Injury is a gigantic public health problem, although it is not conventionally thought of the way we think of cancer or heart disease or infectious diseases," Kellermann said. "You may be in great shape, a nonsmoker, and eat the right foods. But before five o'clock tonight [you or I could] be dead or permanently disabled from an event the public considers an 'accident.' However, there's really no such thing as an accident. Injuries affect high-risk groups and follow an often-predictable chain of events—as surely as lung cancer and heart disease follow smoking. Public health has taught us that any adverse health event that is predictable is also preventable. It's that simple."

And this is where the public health approach to violence becomes interesting and *useful*. From where I stand in the emergency department, a gunshot wound is an injury to treat and a life to save. For a public health doctor like Dr. Yasmin, evaluating a single gunshot victim requires taking a step back. Never taking her eye off the patient, her approach would be to take a holistic assessment of who the person is, where they live, and what their whole life really looks like. Her goal is to provide the maximum benefit for the largest number of patients and to answer the question, What life circumstances and events led to this patient arriving in the emergency department today and what could we have done along the way to prevent them from ever crossing the path of a bullet?

Yasmin might think of gun violence as analogous to an infectious disease. A virus, such as SARS-CoV-2, which causes COVID-19, spreads from one person to the next and the next, causing sickness as it is transmitted (see fig. 2.1). With an outbreak of infection, she would seek to break that *chain of transmission*—what those in the injury prevention world term *the cycle of violence*—and prevent the pathogen spreading from one person to another. Consider for just a few seconds: What is the pathogen, or infectious agent, behind firearm injuries and deaths?

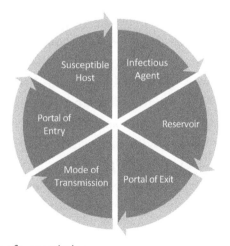

FIGURE 2.1   Chain of transmission

The epidemiologist, or disease detective, would investigate and intervene in the spread of infectious diseases by using tools such as disease surveillance systems, contact tracing, patient education, nonpharmacologic interventions (e.g., masks), or pharmacologic interventions (e.g., vaccines). She can do the same for gun violence using a similar approach. First, she finds out who is getting hurt, then she investigates who is hurting them, where the shooting is happening, and how widespread the problem is. Second, she works to figure out why shootings are occurring and what worsens the problem or improves it. Third, she designs interventions that could prevent gun violence. And finally, she tests her interventions in different settings and studies them to find what works and what doesn't.

The public health approach to gun violence is familiar to practitioners such as Dr. Gary Slutkin, an epidemiologist and infectious disease control specialist who, after tackling HIV, tuberculosis, and cholera around the world for more than two decades, decided that the same infection control approach could be used to counter gun violence.

In the mid-1990s, Slutkin began a program called CeaseFire that trained members of Chicago communities to counter the violence threatening their neighborhoods. "Outsiders can guide and train and provide people with skills," Slutkin told the *New York Times*, "But all epidemics are always worked from the inside out."[5] His program, renamed Cure Violence, trains community members to be "violence interrupters" in their own neighborhoods. Tasked with seeking out encounters that are soon to turn violent, the violence interrupters carefully talk people out of using a gun to settle a dispute—an intervention that can break an entire chain of transmission, since one shooting can set off a cycle of violence that culminates in retaliatory attacks.

Cure Violence, housed at the University of Illinois at Chicago School of Public Health, declared its roots in the public health approach to violence control, but it isn't the city's first peer-education violence-prevention organization. In the 1940s, so-called street work was used to mitigate violence and protect the peace on the streets of Chicago. Cure Violence professionalized and scaled up the approach and aligned it with public health values. After finding success in Chicago, Slutkin's team expanded its model to the Middle East, North Africa, and Latin America.

The city of San Pedro Sula, Honduras, is considered the most violent place on earth. It has a murder rate 31 times the global average. San Pedro Sula implemented this approach to violence prevention and has seen success. In parts of the city where Cure Violence has trained violence interrupters and implemented a public health approach to violence, some communities have gone for 17 months without a single shooting.[6]

The infectious disease analogy for the transmission of gun violence is useful in thinking about the root causes of gun violence, but it poses a tricky question. Take malaria, an infectious disease that kills one child worldwide every two minutes and takes nearly half a million lives globally each year.[7] When you think of malaria, you might think first of mosquitoes, but malaria isn't *caused* by mosquitoes—it's only *spread* by them. The actual cause of the disease malaria is a microscopic parasite called plasmodium that lives in the stomach and salivary glands of the mosquitoes that inject these parasites into humans when they take a drink of blood.

Mosquitoes are the *vectors* of disease; the plasmodium parasite is the causative *agent*, the thing that causes someone to convulse and seize and die from malaria. I view guns like mosquitoes: they are the vectors that help inflict damage, but they are not the root cause of disease. The causative agents are anger, racism, misogyny, suicidality and hate—a sense of hopelessness, a feeling that the problems at hand cannot be fixed with anything other than violence.

These problems are rooted in the factors the disease detectives identified in places that experience outbursts of violence: discrimination such as racism and classism, trauma from child abuse, unemployment, poor education, and failing social welfare systems, all of which can lead to scenarios in which a person armed with a gun sees the bullet as their best available option for fixing a problem. This leads to a bigger conversation about caring for the most vulnerable in society, fostering humanity, and deepening understanding in a polarized society, all of which might take the emphasis away from the gun while focusing on the series of life events that led a person to pick up a gun and use it as a problem solver in the first place.

Some Americans argue that the answer is to take guns out of the equation altogether. I don't think this is a feasible option in the United States, where the right to bear arms is baked into our Constitution—and our cultural identity. There are more guns in America than there are Americans.

Others say that applying the language of public health undermines efforts to stop gun violence, that the word epidemic conjures up natural disasters and plagues, an effect that might promote a narrative of helplessness while absolving humans of responsibility. I disagree.

American's gun fever has contributed to an endemic crisis of violence. What we see in the form of gun violence in the United States is an anomaly to the rest of the world. In 2020, over 45,000 Americans died, and on average over 80,000 Americans are injured by guns annually. This is our baseline, our not-so-new normal. Even for emergency physicians and trauma surgeons accustomed to treating acute symptoms and staunching the flow of blood, the public health approach offers an evidence-based way to rethink this crisis, to treat the root causes in homes and neighborhoods instead of only resorting to patching up the injured on the job. The public health approach could keep gunshot patients out of our nation's emergency departments and trauma bays altogether.

The public health approach can work in cities such as Chicago and Baltimore and around the world.[8] But like Dr. Li Wenliang ringing the alarm about COVID-19 as a new virus surged through his hospital in China, too many are ignoring the cries of those who want to apply this innovative approach to gun violence. For me, it's not about blame or removing guns, it's about mapping the problem, finding root causes, helping those at risk so they don't hurt another person; it's about breaking the chain of transmission and stopping the cycle of violence.

The right treatment for a condition requires a correct diagnosis, and the very first step requires employing the proven public health approach. This is where everything fell apart in the United States. Physicians and research scientists found a critical link in the chain of infection for gun violence, but following this discovery, major antagonists—the National Rifle Association in particular—lobbied to block researchers from continuing to collect data, leaving us stuck in a loop of escalating violence. Preventing scientists from studying gun violence keeps us at a stalemate, even while a proven remedy could help. Why would anybody want to block that? In the next chapter, we investigate why the money hungry and those driven by power worked to block research that could have prevented hundreds of thousands of deaths and injuries. Beyond that investigation, we offer solutions from an emergency medicine doctor and a public health doctor that could break the cycle that has led to gun violence becoming synonymous with the American way of life—and death.

CHAPTER THREE

What's Going On?

"If you got something to say, you better do it in person!" Gaye screamed from his bedroom, incensed that his father was again arguing with his mother Alberta over some misplaced insurance document. The older man, whose receding hair was peppered with blotches of gray, ignored his son's taunt initially. Then, in a huff, he bounded up the stairs toward his son's room, where Alberta had sought refuge from the verbal assault of her husband.

Hearing the footfalls grow louder and louder on the stairs, Gaye bolted to his bedroom door. "Get out of here!" he exclaimed. His father, an overbearing man who had doled out brutal whippings on his son when growing up and had loomed as a feared figure in the eyes of his children, now stood face-to-face with Marvin Gaye, the internationally famous soul singer, who was living with his parents in their home in Los Angeles. Blocking the door, protecting his mother who hid inside his room, Marvin, clad in a maroon house robe, went on the offensive, pushing his father out of the doorway. Marvin's pupils dilated as adrenaline surged with his growing rage. Knowing that his father had always warned that his children should never lay hands on him, Marvin decided that now was the time—he yielded to his anger, punching and kicking his father back down the stairs.

Alberta peered out of the room, watching as Marvin brutally kicked his father. She had to stop him or he might kill him. After all, he was still her husband, despite the abuse and the incessant arguments over those misplaced papers. "Stop!" Alberta shouted to her son. It was no use: Marvin was beyond reason as he fought back against his father. Alberta ran down the stairs, pulled Marvin away, and ushered him back up to his bedroom. Sweating, panting to catch his breath, he stood there, silent.

Then, footfalls.

Marvin's father was returning up the stairs. He burst into the room, displaying a .38 caliber pistol, and quietly pulled the trigger. Marvin screamed when the first shot struck him. Alberta wanted to run but couldn't. Her attention was transfixed on her son, who slid down to the floor. Marvin's father walked closer and pulled the trigger again. With the entrance to the room now vacated and Marvin Sr. standing over his son, Alberta ran out of the house, fearful for her own life. Her other son, Frankie, and his wife, Irene, caught her outside.

"He's shot Marvin," she said. "He's killed my boy."

Frankie ventured inside, went up the stairs, and found Marvin laying in a pool of blood. Looking up with an unexpectedly sallow face, Marvin whispered to his brother, "I got what I wanted. I couldn't do it myself, so I had him do it." Marvin had been struggling again with drugs and with depression. "It's good, I ran my race," he told his brother. "There's no more left in me." Marvin Gaye died the day before his 45th birthday by the gun he had given to his father just a few months before at Christmas.

***

Arthur "Art" Kellermann, a 29-year-old physician, looked up from his epidemiology textbook when the news crashed over the radio. He caught the eyes of one of his classmates who was staring back at him and muttered, "This is nuts." At the time, in April 1984, he was at the University of Washington, studying public health.

Kellermann, a tall, lanky man with a distinct country drawl, had been inspired to become a doctor after shadowing Dr. Hiram Moore, his father's best friend since childhood, in South Pittsburgh, Tennessee, during the early 1970s. Moore was a Black physician who began his medical practice in the segregated South in the late 1940s. Shadowing Moore one day on his hospital rounds, a young Kellermann confided that his chances of getting into medical school were slim because of his poor freshman grades at Rhodes College.

Moore challenged him. Conversations that summer between the young student and the veteran doctor motivated Kellermann to stop dwelling on poor grades and to focus on learning the skills doctors relied on day-to-day. Kellermann threw himself into learning how to give injections and take X-rays. He ran back and forth between the ward and the lab, realizing that a career in medicine relied on teamwork and practical skills.

Kellermann eventually made it to medical school, graduating from Emory University in Atlanta, Georgia, before heading west to do an internal medicine residency at the University of Washington in Seattle. He trained as an emergency room doctor but became interested in public health. Therefore, he signed up for the Robert Wood Johnson Foundation Clinical Scholars program, a preeminent training program for clinicians interested in a research career. He was in that program when he heard the news about Marvin Gaye.

Gaye's murder prompted Kellermann to think about gun violence not only as an emergency room issue but also as a public health dilemma. Kellermann spoke to his friend over the murmurings of the radio, "There are all these guns in houses, a lot of them are kept for protection, and yet it seems like every other day you hear about somebody shooting their wife, or a son gets shot by his father. Surely somebody has looked at a gun in the home as a risk factor or a protection factor for violent death."

Nobody had.

When he went to the library and combed the medical literature, all Kellermann could find was a passing mention buried in an old issue of a journal; a single sentence that said that keeping a gun in the house for self-defense was more likely to end in the death of a family member than in the death of an intruder. "I saw that observation quoted repeatedly in subsequent editorials or medical reviews but no additional research on the question." So the young doctor got to work.

First, Kellermann tracked down everyone who had died from a bullet in the Seattle, Washington, area from 1978 to 1983. Piecing together clues from police files and autopsy reports, Kellermann studied the murderers, their victims, and the sordid details of their dying moments. He tallied 743 people who had been killed by a bullet in Seattle over those six years. Half of the victims had been killed in their own homes, where they had kept a gun. By parsing the data, Kellermann calculated that there were thirty-seven times as many suicides in homes with a gun and almost five times as many gun deaths in homes with a firearm than in homes without one.

Kellermann published his research in 1986 in one of medicine's most prestigious journals, the *New England Journal of Medicine*. His concluding line made a bold statement: "The advisability of keeping firearms in the home for protection must be questioned."[1]

Kellermann then took a closer look at Vancouver, Canada, a three-hour drive away. Vancouver was like Seattle in many ways, but it had taken a stricter approach to gun regulation. He compared gun violence in both cities and found that while Seattle and Vancouver had similar rates of robberies and burglaries, people in Seattle were seven times more likely to experience assault involving a gun than their neighbors north of the border. In fact, a Seattle resident's likelihood of being shot to death was almost five times higher than that of a resident of Vancouver. Kellermann concluded that stricter gun regulation could reduce the murder rate.

In 1993, Kellermann returned to Emory University, where he had attended medical school, to establish the Emory Center for Injury Control at Rollins School of Public Health. As an emergency physician, Kellermann had a vested interest in studying violence and preventing injury. "It became increasingly apparent to me that no matter how well we ran the emergency department, no matter how well we taught residents, until we address fundamental social and medical issues that are affecting our society and learn how we can better prevent injuries and other major health problems . . . we're not going to get a handle on this problem."

His approach was this: use the tools of public health to combat injuries caused by firearms. The same year that he launched the Center for Injury Control, Kellermann published the findings of a long and arduous research project that involved months of combing through the records of every single person murdered in their homes in King County, Washington; Shelby County, Tennessee; and Cuyahoga County, Ohio, from 1987 to 1992.

Researchers such as Kellermann use epidemiological techniques to keep us safer by investigating what causes illness, but it can be difficult to find the root cause in some cases. They have several ways of looking at a problem to tease out cause and correlation in order to answer the following questions: Did A cause B or would B have happened anyway? Or did A increase the likelihood of B occurring? Causality means that because of A, B happened, whereas correlation only implies that linkage.

Kellermann used a specific method for his research called a case-control study, one that compares people who have a disease—the cases—to people who do not have the disease—the controls. To be accurate, controls must be like the cases in almost every other way. He compared the cases to the controls to see if an exposure—to guns, in this case—was related to an outcome, death. It was.

We need to be careful with our words here: *related* is different than saying something *caused* another thing to happen. I'm sure you've heard the phrase *correlation is not causation*, and case-control studies cannot prove that one thing caused another. But they can show us if and how strongly two things are connected. Looking at the death records from the three counties, Kellermann and his team identified close to 2,000 people who had been murdered and found that around one in four victims had been murdered in their homes. Around one in ten was murdered outside their home but within the property lines.

Most murders played out like this: a person was embroiled in an argument—or what Kellermann described as "a romantic triangle"—with someone they knew well, perhaps a lover or family member, and in the heat of the argument, that person used a gun to kill them. Kellermann concluded that people who kept a gun in their homes were almost three times more likely to be murdered than a person who did not keep a gun. This study established the link between keeping a gun in the house and being murdered by someone you know.

Yet when I interviewed him, Kellermann refused to describe himself as either pro-gun or anti-gun. He grew up with guns and enjoyed shooting them as a boy in rural Tennessee. Now a man in his late sixties who was the chief executive officer of the Virginia Commonwealth University Health System until November 2022, he has dedicated much of his life to studying things other than guns. If you look up his extensive body of research, you'll find that the majority of Kellermann's published studies are not about guns; they are research studies about heart attacks, high blood pressure, military medicine, and cardiopulmonary resuscitation. Kellermann sees all these ailments, and guns, as connected to America's health.

***

For close to two decades, I have similarly found myself at the crossroads between the two worlds—public health and private medicine—that Kellermann straddled over the expanse of his career. One day, during the third year of my time at New York University School of Medicine, the year when we finally got a chance to roam the hospital wards, I saw a flyer in the dean's office about a scholarship to earn a public health degree from Columbia University, a nearby institution on the Upper West Side of New York City. I rolled the dice, took my shot, and was accepted to the program.

Two decades later, I sit at this strange and often uncomfortable nexus where I know more than the average physician about certain health policy issues and more than the average policy wonk about standing at the bedside of a bleeding gunshot victim. I have fervently come to believe that the role of the physician does not end at the bedside. In fact, training in public health and health policy taught me to think about not just the person immediately in front of me but also all the other people who I might never meet but whose lives I could powerfully impact through health policies made at the hospital, city, county, state, or federal levels.

My thinking was formed through classroom instruction on city management from David Dinkins, the first Black mayor of New York City, and during the summer of 2005 from my service as a staff assistant in the House of Representatives, where I worked for the Ways and Means Committee under ranking member Charlie Rangel. On Capitol Hill, I realized the greater impact that public health and health policy can have on my patients and their communities than whatever I scribble onto a prescription pad.

A few years ago, I wanted to illustrate this fact to a group of young emergency medicine residents—physicians who, after graduating medical school, train in the specialty of emergency medicine. Using back-of-the-envelope calculations, I demonstrated the importance of incorporating the concepts of public health, policy, and advocacy into their careers. I asked them, "How many people's lives will the average emergency physician impact?" They had never even considered quantifying their career by its impact on other human beings.

I did the math for them.

The average emergency physician who works a standard job in a community emergency department will see at least two patients per hour; that's approximately 2,880 patients each year. Next, I asked the trainees to calculate, as a comparison, how many peoples' lives President Barack Obama touched when he signed the Affordable Care Act into law in 2010. With the stroke of his pen, Obama extended health coverage to over 22 million Americans in the act's first few years of existence. Using data from a similar health care coverage expansion in Massachusetts, research has revealed an interesting fact—for every 830 people who gained insurance, one life was saved.[2]

So what happens when we extrapolate that number on a national scale using President Obama's signature health care law? It would take the average emergency physician over eight years to save as many lives as Barack Obama did when he signed the Affordable Care Act into law. And despite what you might see on the television, for most of the patients we see every day in the emergency department, physicians are not intervening in a way that is significant enough to save a life. Truthfully, we see a fair number of stubbed toes and medication refills and not just heart attacks, strokes, and trauma victims all day.

Even if we could boast that we saved the lives of one out of every three people we treated, it would take the average emergency physician roughly a full career to save as many lives as President Obama saved with his most lasting, signature achievement in office. As Joe Biden whispered into Obama's ear the day that bill was signed, the Affordable Care Act was indeed a "big fucking deal."

I present this argument to young physicians and medical students when explaining to them why I believe that it is critical that they learn to advocate on behalf of their patients, both individually at the bedside and collectively in the political arena, so that we can save as many lives as possible. Some will be those on whom we lay hands, others we will never personally know. This is a lesson I have learned from studying the life of Dr. Kellermann: when you find a problem in society, you tackle it not by political means but through scientific ones. In this case, that's where public health and research comes into play. Public health describes the problem. Its methods can be used to analyze potential solutions to the problem. And with these solutions in hand, people can advocate for the best means to change our society for the better. Would Marvin Gaye still be alive if he or his family knew that having a gun in the home was more likely to cause harm than to be used for protection? The trauma Gaye suffered—and the trauma of those who suffered vicariously through his death—can be used for good. It helped someone like Kellermann contemplate what's going on in our society and uncover opportunities to impact our communities for the better. Unfortunately, organizations like the National Rifle Association would look at the data presented by Dr. Kellermann and would revolt against science instead of heeding its warnings.

CHAPTER FOUR

The Revolt against Science

Summer arrived swiftly in Cincinnati in 1977, with temperatures surpassing eighty degrees and lovers pressing clammy hands together as Marvin Gaye's live recording of "Got to Give It Up" melted out of radio speakers in the Midwestern city on the Ohio River.

Gaye's falsetto soared across the airwaves as 30,000 gun owners flocked to the Queen City to attend the National Rifle Association's annual meeting in May that year. Founded in 1871 in the aftermath of the Civil War as former generals lamented that Union soldiers couldn't hit the broad side of a barn, the NRA was originally born to improve marksmanship. Its first president was Union general Ambrose Burnside, who had fought in the Battle of Antietam—the bloodiest day in American military history. More than a hundred years later, the 1977 convention in Cincinnati altered the course of the NRA forever.

Former NRA president Harlon Carter arrived in Cincinnati with a contingent of agitators clad in orange hunters' caps. They roamed the convention floor, arguing that the NRA should focus more on its political ambitions. That's where the real influence was, they argued.

For its first 100 years, the NRA behaved differently from the organization Americans know today: it *supported* regulation and restrictions on firearms. Testifying before Congress in 1938, Karl Frederick, the NRA president at that time and a former Olympic sport shooter, supported the first national firearms law, the Federal Firearms Act of 1938, stating, "I do not believe in the general promiscuous toting of guns. I think it should be sharply restricted and only under licenses."[1]

After the assassination of President John F. Kennedy in 1963, the NRA favored regulations to restrict gun purchases and to create federal firearms licensing for gun dealers. And when two dozen members of the Black Panther Party demonstrated at the California capitol while openly carrying rifles in the spring of 1967, the NRA once again supported laws that banned the brandishing of loaded weapons in public. The Mulford Act, signed into law by Governor Ronald Reagan, prohibited the public carry of loaded firearms without a permit in California.

Ten years later, Carter convinced delegates to radically alter the focus of the NRA at an event dubbed the "Revolt at Cincinnati." Although it had not previously been focused on expanding the reach of the Second Amendment, the NRA under Carter's command would no longer compromise when defending Americans' right to bear arms. "There will be no more civil war within the National Rifle Association," Carter said after the power grab.[2] The Revolt at Cincinnati would go largely unnoticed for decades, until the NRA—now detached from its original purpose to "promote and encourage rifle shooting on a scientific basis"[3]—would come across a new foe in the form of academics and physicians such as Dr. Art Kellermann.

***

For hundreds of years, physicians have cared for those injured by guns. Among the 30 million scientific publications in the National Library of Medicine's PubMed database, one of the earliest tales dates to 1820; it describes the surgical repair of a soldier whose jaw was shattered after he was shot in the neck. The bullet exploded out of the other side of his face through the poor man's cheek.[4] Other nineteenth-century stories in the medical literature describe soldiers who, although shot, did not realize it; the pain from the gunshot wounds was little more than what they would have expected if another soldier had accidentally cut them with a sword.[5] The seemingly trivial nature of many gunshot wounds was evident in a depiction of a soldier in the 1880s who thought the man behind him had pricked him in the back and turned around to investigate, only to see his compatriot fall dead to the ground from a bullet wound to the head. Only afterward did the soldier realize that the fatal bullet had first entered his own neck and then exited his back prior to striking and killing the person marching behind him.

A civilian tale from medical examiner Dr. Paul Swift in Philadelphia in 1847 describes a child who was shot by "a minor, [who] playfully, but heedlessly, fired a pistol charged with powder only, at his friend and companion."[6] The child died. But it was far from immediate. Instead, the child suffered a slow and painful death from a tetanus infection, the result of the dirty wadding that riddled his body.

These stories, memories of a distant past preserved on fading paper—now scanned into digital documents—represent just one-quarter of one-tenth of 1% of all the medical literature that exists. This miniscule fraction is the research that contains the word "firearm."[7] Studying the effects of human firearm injuries and deaths would not be prominent again until many decades later. A *New England Journal of Medicine* article from 1977, the same year as the Revolt at Cincinnati, described the changing pattern of homicides in metropolitan Cleveland, Ohio, during 1958–1974, noting "a conspicuous rise in firearm killings."[8] Those researchers noted that homicide was a major cause of death for young, urban, non-white men and that there was a startling link to handgun use. Fifty years later, those demographics haven't changed much.

Compared to a century earlier, when doctors essentially traded watercooler stories about soldiers who were shot in combat, physicians and academics nowadays use scientific methods and public health strategies to formally study the human toll of guns. Or at least they try to, when political pressures do not impede the flow of science.

Art Kellermann was among the first to champion public health strategies to evaluate firearm injuries and deaths. He is quick to point out the many others engaged in such research, such as pediatrician Fred Rivara, with whom Kellermann has published copious research on firearm homicides.[9]

Other physicians, such as Dr. David Brent, focused on gun-related suicides. Suicide remains the foremost cause of firearm deaths in the United States by a margin of nearly two to one. Brent, a psychiatrist, discovered that major risk factors among teens—such as a diagnosis of either bipolar disorder or affective disorder, a lack of prior treatment for mental health issues, and the availability of firearms in the home—explained a large majority of the difference between life and death for these adolescents.[10] While a mental health disorder might serve as a risk factor for suicide by gun, it is by no means a guarantee that a person will die from suicide, just as diabetes is a risk factor for but not a guarantee of a future heart attack.

Still, many assume that people with mental health issues can simply control their problem with sheer willpower. You can't tell someone to "be stronger" and eliminate their mental health issues, any more than you can tell someone with diabetes to command their pancreas to churn out more insulin.

I once cared for a teenager who was feeling withdrawn and suicidal. He believed that if he was "stronger" his depression would abate. As I walked out of the examination room, I explained to my resident trainee what care the patient needed, including psychotherapy and medications. But I also mentioned the need to talk about guns. As physicians, we must talk with our patients (and our politicians) about keeping firearms in the home and how this can impact the lives of the most vulnerable.

While Kellermann's research showed that having a gun in the home increased the risk of homicide by nearly three times, Brent's studies found that having any type of gun in the home more than quadrupled the risk of suicide among teens irrespective of whether a previous psychiatric condition was present.[11] If the firearm was a handgun, the risk of suicide increased more than nine times. For teens without preexisting mental health disorders, a loaded weapon in the home increased the risk of suicide more than 32 times. These data moved Brent and his colleagues to say that prevention of suicide in teens without preexisting mental health disorders is "probably best achieved by restriction of the availability of firearms, particularly loaded ones."[12]

The strong link between the availability of a gun and death by gunshot has led injury prevention experts to focus on a concept known as *means restriction*. Realizing that someone who intends to kill themself has many different options—such as using a ligature (like a rope) or medication (like sedatives)—it makes sense to restrict the most lethal means of doing harm. And a gun, after all, is a very efficient way to end a life. Compared to attempted hangings, where over 50% of people succeed, and ingestions of pills, where fewer than 2% of attempts end in death, nearly 90% who attempt suicide by gun die.[13]

Standing inside my Houston emergency department on an especially hot and humid summer day, I asked a middle-aged white man why he had sought refuge inside the frigid confines of the emergency department. He pulled a thin white sheet up over his shoulders, leaving just his head visible on the stretcher as he told me about his alcohol addiction and how he drank four bottles of wine a day. He was suicidal. He told me that if he could take a single pill and fall asleep forever, he would do it; he would kill himself. As has become part of my routine, I asked him if he had access to a gun.

"I'm too much of a wuss to do that," he replied tearfully.

For those with the intention to die by suicide, guns are the most dangerous of instruments. Means restriction—finding a way to keep guns out of the hands of profoundly suicidal people—saves lives.

The emergency physician and researcher Dr. Garen Wintemute from the UC Davis Medical Center also began his foray into gun violence research in the 1980s. He and his colleagues documented who was most hurt in this uniquely American epidemic.[14] One key demographic was Black men aged 25 to 34 years, who had the highest gun homicide rates. Eight out of ten Black men who died by a bullet were gunned down in a homicide.

Violence like this, the culmination of a conflict between two people who might be strangers, loose acquaintances, or lovers, overwhelmingly represents the type of gun injuries and deaths that I see every day. Wintemute, recognizing the strong connection between the easy availability of guns and gun violence, wrote: "Firearms are hazardous consumer products but are not addressed as such by our current regulatory structure."[15] Wintemute's public support for specific gun control positions pricked up the ears of NRA insiders.[16] The gun lobby, now poised to attack anything that might limit the proliferation of guns in America, had taken notice of the science and could no longer afford to allow physicians, given our trusted position in society, to cast aspersions on guns.

***

When bullets puncture the skin, the kinetic energy from the projectile dissipates into the tissues of the body it strikes, whether that is skin, fat, muscle, solid organs, or bones. As the bullet is slowed by meeting with flesh, it creates a shock wave that is massively larger in size than the bullet itself. This shock wave distorts, twists, and snaps blood vessels, ligaments, and nerves, even those not directly in the path of the bullet. We call this shock wave phenomenon *cavitation*. Cavitation amplifies the damage of a single bullet. It makes firearms a serious threat beyond what someone might observe just by looking at the number of holes left in a punctured body.

Confronted with these injury patterns in his emergency room, Kellermann and his colleagues laid out an aggressive agenda for gun research, including ways to prevent gun injuries and death using the public health approaches of primary, secondary, and tertiary prevention. But the NRA, emboldened after the Revolt at Cincinnati, went on the political offensive. It chose Kellermann as its scapegoat, attacking the science and the scientists who had proven that firearms were more dangerous than Americans had been led to believe. At the urging of the NRA, the US House of Representatives made attempts to strike back at who was funding Kellerman's research—the National Center for Injury Prevention and Control at the Centers for Disease Control and Prevention (CDC). The NRA had hoped to eliminate the center altogether; it failed at that. However, the House of Representatives, controlled by Republican Newt Gingrich as speaker, zeroed out the total amount of money the CDC had spent on gun injury prevention research the prior year in the appropriations bill then under consideration. The funding was later restored in a conference committee with the Senate. But damaging language that admonished the CDC in the final 1996 Omnibus Consolidated Appropriations Act had a damning and decades-long impact on American gun violence research. A phrase that Arkansas Republican Jay Dickey inserted in the law stated that "none of the funds made available for injury prevention and control at the Centers for Disease Control and Prevention may be used to advocate or promote gun control." And just like that, a major source of federal funding for firearm research disappeared. The Dickey Amendment meant that the $2.6 million used for gun violence research by the CDC in the prior year was no longer available to researchers after 1996.

Over the years, researchers lost a cumulative $65 million in funding—$83 million in 2020 dollars adjusted for inflation. This of course assumes there never would have been an increase in the annual appropriation beyond the rate of inflation, a dubious assumption considering the crisis that gun violence proved to be in the following decades.

The Dickey Amendment didn't technically ban gun violence research, but its vagueness left it open to broad interpretation. "Precisely what was or was not permitted under the clause was unclear," Kellermann said. "But no federal employee was willing to risk his or her career or the agency's funding to find out."[17] To Kellerman, the interference of the NRA, while likely not the first attempt by a special-interest group to hamper the work of a public health agency such as the CDC (Big Tobacco is *the* prime example) was "arguably the most egregious" with its effort to thwart scientific truth.[18]

After his retirement from Congress, Jay Dickey grew to regret his role in the NRA's campaign against science. In 2015, he wrote a letter to Member of Congress Mike Thompson, chair of an important committee in the House of Representatives, that said that "research could have been continued on gun violence without infringing on the rights of gun owners, in the same fashion that the highway industry continued its research without eliminating the automobile."[19]

Science is a process through which researchers try to find truth, or at least come close to it. The public has seen the scientific process play out in real time during the COVID pandemic. It's messy. Scientists might publicly disagree with one another. One set of studies finds holes in others, depending on the methods involved and the populations studied. This can make it challenging to come up with real-world solutions while revealing to the public the fact that science is not simply a bunch of facts; science is a process, often a complex and contradictory one. And even when the facts can be agreed upon, the same results might be interpreted quite differently by two different researchers, based on their expertise and personal biases.

But the gun lobby was unwilling to even engage with this nuanced viewpoint. Its stance: kill the science altogether. With the Dickey Amendment, the NRA won a major battle in the war against science, the war against public health, and the war against truth. Much like the pandemic-era fight against wearing face masks to prevent the spread of COVID-19, the NRA had succeeded in politicizing the public health approach and polarizing the public.

Scientific advances in medicine, aeronautics, atomic energy, telecommunications, and other areas had defined America in the twentieth century. But for the first time, the blood supply of potentially lifesaving public health research had been stanched. At the urgings of an organization focused on allowing more firearms to enter the homes of American consumers, the American public was left without data about who had been injured or killed by firearms and when, how, and where that had happened.

CHAPTER FIVE

Canary in the Coal Mine

Worldwide, three of out every ten women experience intimate partner violence in their lifetime.[1] In the United States, the presence of a gun in these situations increases the risk of death by over five times.[2] Unaware of those facts, a young woman from western New York rode her bicycle from a village in Côte d'Ivoire down a worn path to a small town 90 minutes away. Sweating heavily, she arrived at one of the few shops in the area with air conditioning. Leaving the bike on the stoop, its back wheel slowly spinning as it lay on its side, she sat down inside the shop and waited for the sweat to crystallize into salt on her pale skin. Only then did she pull out pen and paper from her backpack to start scribbling out her name and address information about her education and other details about her life.

Megan Ranney, an affable American woman who was a freshly minted graduate of Harvard University with a degree in the history of science, thought her path forward would be as a journalist perhaps, or doing what she was doing in the late 1990s, working in West Africa as a humanitarian for the Peace Corps. Officially there to help with access to clean water and sanitation, Ranney soon discovered that the greatest need was for help with a new contagion, human immunodeficiency virus (HIV). The virus weakened the immune system, making people vulnerable to infections that a healthy body could fight. But one of the biggest problems wasn't the virus itself; it was the stigma surrounding those who were infected and the violence that had led to a propagating epidemic.

"Without talking about the infection, there was no way to prevent its spread," Ranney later reflected when recalling her experiences in that small village in the middle of a nation with a population roughly the size of Texas. Ranney wanted to tell the stories of the villagers she now knew as neighbors, detailing the patterns of disease and injuries they faced in their daily struggle to exist on less than one dollar a day. But after learning about friend after friend becoming infected with HIV, many at the hands of abusive spouses, she could no longer tell their stories of intimate partner violence without wanting to intervene.

That day in the shop, while cooling off from the Ivorian sun, Ranney wrote applications for medical school. She had made this trek to the air-conditioned shop specifically so that sweat would not stain the pages of crisp white paper she would mail back to the United States. In her applications and essays to admissions committees at American medical schools, Ranney described her experience with the Peace Corps.

"I lived in a small village in the center of Côte d'Ivoire, where no one spoke English and few spoke French," she later explained. "I had no running water or electricity. My official job was to improve water and sanitation, but I ended up spending most of my time on HIV prevention, focusing on the destigmatization of the disease and discussions of the drivers of disease. No one would even admit that they, or a family member, were infected with HIV."

She spent countless hours talking about sexual assault and domestic violence, including to many women who over weeks would become her friends. "At that time, in that country, it was an unusual topic to discuss," she explained. "I worked with a number of local and regional community groups to start community-level conversations about condom use and sexual violence, among other preventive measures."

Her time in Africa was transformative. She drifted across that imaginary line separating public health and private medical care. While Ranney had intended to live in the public health sphere, she now felt the calling to become a physician. Others, having learned the art and science of medicine first, eventually realized that the care of people other than just the patient sitting across from you eventually necessitates a public health approach. Physicians such as Ranney and I walk the same path, skilled clinicians capable of dealing with each patient one-on-one but also focused on improving the health of communities and entire nations.

Ranney enrolled at Columbia University's College of Physicians and Surgeons, a prestigious institution housed in the stately complex of brown brick buildings in Manhattan's Washington Heights neighborhood. Then, after graduating with numerous honors, she left New York for Providence, Rhode Island, to begin a career at Brown University in emergency medicine. Ranney chose emergency medicine "because it is, to me, the best place in our health system to help people through the public health approach. We see everyone, regardless of ability to pay, education, immigration status, or any other social marker. We are the canary in the coal mine for societal epidemics. We have the potential to identify problems—and implement change—in a really unique way." Her reasons sound a lot like the admonition of the nineteenth-century physician, Rudolf

Virchow, who argued that physicians should deal with the problems of society as a whole and not just the patient in front of them. Virchow believed that "medicine, as a social science, as the science of human beings, has the obligation to point out problems and to attempt their theoretical solution."[3]

When she began her emergency medicine residency program, Ranney thought she might follow Virchow's path of social medicine with a foray into a global health. It made sense. She already had experience working internationally, and the profession of emergency medicine imbues its practitioners with a broad skill set that lends perfectly to work in under-resourced or underserved locales. During her residency program, Ranney spent a significant portion of her time in western Kenya working on the prevention of gender-based violence—the same violence she had witnessed in Côte d'Ivoire during the years before she entered medical school. She remarked that she "was there at the same time that [Kenya] was passing its first laws making rape a crime."[4] But instead of global health, Ranney realized that the current underlying her passion happened to be violence. So instead of traveling the world again, she stayed in Rhode Island.

"I had committed to a fellowship in injury prevention to learn the science behind domestic violence and sexual assault prevention," she says. "It was only later that I transitioned to focusing on community violence and gun violence." That transition began for Ranney after she witnessed a few tragic cases in which domestic violence intersected with firearm violence.

But even before Ranney had started her fellowship, the NRA had begun to work against her and others who wanted to pursue injury prevention as a career. The NRA's silencing of the science of firearm injury prevention at the CDC had already been in force for twelve years. The funding that had previously been available to the injury prevention community now came with dire warning to avoid "advocacy." Ranney remains especially cautious when speaking so that people won't mistake her work to promote unbiased research as advocacy for gun control.

But what exactly is advocacy? Is a scientist researching a topic being an advocate? Does the moniker fit if we tell the public about the findings of such research? Or does it only become advocacy when we mention the science to our politicians? The ambiguity of that answer meant that millions of dollars had evaporated by the time Ranney and her contemporaries were coming of age and creating their own niches in the injury prevention space. She and others had even been advised by mentors to avoid the subject of gun violence altogether.

But Ranney was stubborn. She was determined to become strictly a researcher, not an advocate, so as to avoid the ire of potential funders. During her fellowship, another study came out that linked firearm ownership with gun assaults. This case-control study based in Philadelphia reported that "individuals in possession of a gun were 4.46 times more likely to be shot in an assault than those not in possession."[5] Again, the science directly contradicted the narrative from the NRA, one that Wayne LaPierre, the NRA's front man in 2012, articulated as "the only way to stop a bad guy with a gun is with a good guy with a gun." According to the accumulated facts, however, it seemed that the good guy was simply more likely to be shot by the bad guy.

The CDC didn't support the study out of Philadelphia financially. Instead the funding came from the National Institute on Alcohol Abuse and Alcoholism at the National Institutes of Health (NIH). Alarmed that science was still threatening to inform the American public about the true dangers of firearms, the NRA successfully lobbied, again, to put in place language restricting the use of federal funds to advocate for gun control in the Consolidated Appropriations Act of 2012, effectively killing gun violence research from the NIH.[6] Just like it had with the Dickey Amendment, the NRA had found a powerful means to effectively tie the hands of the scientific community by establishing that any scientific inquiry into the impacts of firearms funded by taxpayer dollars would not be tolerated.

Mark Rosenberg, former director of the CDC's National Center for Injury Control and Prevention, strikingly said that "the scientific community has been terrorized by the NRA," referring to the political tactics it has used to silence the science.[7] Academics who had been active in injury prevention research shifted focus away from firearms into other, more financially viable lines of research. The few that remained would be forced to continue their research using their own personal time and money, an investment not everyone could make, whittling the cohort of firearms researchers to a dedicated few. And soon after the NRA sabotaged the scientific community by limiting NIH funding for firearms research, a madman would terrorize a small town in Connecticut, abruptly propelling the epidemic of gun violence back into the spotlight.

***

A gaunt young man with brown curls sweeping down his face wrapped a long white index finger around the trigger of a .22-caliber Savage Mark II rifle, aiming at the head of his mother while she slept. He squeezed the trigger, sending four blasts careening through her head, murdering Nancy Lanza as she lay asleep in her pajamas. Then the man drove his mother's car to Sandy Hook Elementary School, his mind clouded in a murderous rage.[8] He killed twenty young schoolchildren and six teachers on December 14, 2012, before turning a gun on himself in what, at the time, was one of the worst mass shootings in American history.

President Barack Obama, a parent of two young girls, addressed the nation later that day. "We've endured too many of these tragedies in the past few years," he said. "And each time I learn the news I react not as a President, but as anybody else would—as a parent. And that was especially true today. I know there's not a parent in America who doesn't feel the same overwhelming grief that I do." Standing behind a podium in the White House that bore the seal of the president, he paused for 11 seconds, holding his hand near his left eye as if to hold back tears. President Obama continued his speech, landing a phrase that struck those in the injury prevention community as especially poignant. "We're going to have to come together and take meaningful action to *prevent* more tragedies like this, regardless of the politics."[9]

For many in America, the shooting at Sandy Hook was a turning point in the debate about gun violence. Shannon Watts, the mother of five children, began a conversation the following day through a Facebook page she called One Million Moms for Gun Control. In the aftermath of the killing of twenty children and six schoolteachers, Watts's passion and advocacy eventually evolved into the organization Moms Demand Action, a nonprofit group that a decade later had over 6 million community activists on its rolls.

As a parent herself, Ranney understood the importance of research informing policy. Cautiously, she notes the need for advocates to use unbiased research to inform their pleas to lawmakers. "Policy is part; but policy is not sufficient," Ranney says. For her, it is more important to activate networks of change. While the lack of available funding caused many others to pursue other avenues of research, Ranney continued headlong toward what many of her mentors described to her as a dead end for her career.

But the lack of federal funding did not deter her. Ranney had lived in West Africa without electricity amid sexual violence, stigma, and limited resources to fight valiantly against the HIV epidemic. At a time when many people sat comfortably in their apartments or dorm rooms to apply to medical school, she biked to a nearby village to fill out her applications. She would never retreat from a difficult or even seemingly impossible situation.

After Sandy Hook and the many mass shootings that have followed, Ranney continued to focus her work on injury prevention science by studying firearms as a means of injury. She has chaired the Firearm Injury Policy subcommittee of the American College of Emergency Physicians' Public Health and Injury Prevention Committee and was appointed as the Rhode Island representative to the Multi-state Governor's Work Group on Firearm Injury Research. In 2019, she earned a seat on the Scientific Advisory Committee of the New Jersey Gun Violence Research Center. And because federal funds were essentially nonexistent, she cofounded a nonprofit, the American Foundation for Firearm Injury Reduction in Medicine (AFFIRM), serving as its chief research officer, to fill the void in federal research funding left by the subversive actions of the gun lobby. And she would be prepared for the next time the NRA wanted to take a cheap shot at doctors who wanted to use science to protect their patients.

CHAPTER SIX

This Is Our Lane

On November 7, 2018, the National Rifle Association sent out a tweet criticizing a publication from the American College of Physicians (ACP). The ACP, a professional organization of internal medicine doctors, had recently written a position paper that members believed would help save American lives from the ravages of gun violence.[1] In the years since the NRA sneaked the Dickey Amendment into the budget for the CDC and added a similar rider into that of the NIH, effectively terminating federal research on gun violence, medical organizations continued to use what data existed—as well as commonsense solutions—to improve the lives of their communities and their patients.

My specialty organization, the American College of Emergency Physicians, had long argued for restoring federal funding to firearms injury prevention research and for implementing policies such as universal background checks and bans on assault weapons. But the NRA didn't believe it was the role of physicians to worry about the health hazards of firearms. Whose role is it, then?

Following the Revolt at Cincinnati, the NRA abandoned the first phrase of the Second Amendment, the one that focused on *a well-regulated militia*, and instead concentrated solely on the portion that stated that gun ownership *shall not be infringed*. Feeling that physicians would stand in the way of that objective, the NRA has not only worked to defund research but has also supported gag laws that would prevent pediatricians from asking parents about gun ownership.[2]

The American College of Pediatrics, the American Medical Association, and the ACP successfully sued the state of Florida, which in 2011 passed a law prohibiting physicians from asking parents about guns in the home. Several other physician specialty organizations and the American Bar Association stood aligned in opposition to these types of laws, which prohibit the free speech of physicians and interfere with the doctor-patient relationship.[3]

Following the ACP's 2018 position statement, the NRA shot back at doctors: "Someone should tell self-important anti-gun doctors to stay in their lane. Half of the articles in Annals of Internal Medicine are pushing for gun control. Most upsetting, however, the medical community seems to have consulted NO ONE but themselves."[4]

It was an unseasonably warm autumn afternoon and I was dropping my son off at his grandmother's house in advance of an upcoming overnight shift in the emergency department when I saw that tweet. At first I was dismissive. I thought to myself, "Whatever!" before driving to work. It was absurd for me to believe that the physician's lane ends at the bedside.

What is the physician's lane?

The physician's role includes policy. When I worked with the House Ways and Means Committee as a staffer, I listened to constituents and special-interest groups discuss their policy positions The physician's role includes educating our lawmakers. I learned that nonprofits and other advocacy groups can serve in that role when I was working for the Kaiser Family Foundation while completing my emergency medicine residency in Washington, DC. The physician's lane includes advocacy. I've been on the other end of table—lobbying Capitol Hill staff, state legislators, and even members of Congress—to argue for laws that would be beneficial to my profession and my patients.

The modern NRA has stood in contradiction to everything I had learned as both a physician and as an advocate for public health. Five hours after the NRA's tweet, the House of Medicine would resound with one voice: #ThisIsOurLane.[5]

***

Dr. Abbie Youkilis, a physician who has cared for many survivors of gun violence while working at the Cincinnati Veterans' Affairs Medical Center, had been monitoring the NRA and its spokesperson Dana Loesch intently for several months, ever since her niece, Jaime Guttenberg, had been murdered in the school shooting at Marjory Stoneman Douglas High School in Parkland, Florida. In the months that followed, she had reached out to Megan Ranney, the emergency physician at Brown University, during a parents' weekend; Youkilis's daughter was enrolled there too. When Youkilis saw the NRA's "obnoxious" tweet, as she called it, she tipped off Ranney. As a federal employee, Youkilis felt she couldn't personally be as vocal on the issue as others could, like her brother Fred Guttenberg, Jaime's father. She hoped that people like Ranney could be the voice that she could not.

For years, Ranney had been cataloging the impact of gun violence as witnessed by physicians. She has thousands of stories to tell of these tragedies. She's seen multiple women brought in who had been shot by their partners, often in murder-suicides, some who were pregnant, some who had recently left an abusive relationship, and some whose shooting was meant as a tool of intimidation.

As an injury prevention expert, Ranney had sought to work with firearm owners to solve gun violence in America through public health techniques but had been consistently rebuffed by the gun lobby. Incensed by the continued assault on the firearm injury prevention community, Ranney graciously—far more graciously than I would have been—extended an olive branch in her reaction to the NRA, suggesting, "We can have law-abiding, safe gun owners as part of the conversation about how to reduce gun violence . . . whether or not the NRA chooses to join."[6] Her message, and those of other physicians, nurses, and health care workers, started to flood the internet.

I arrived at work that night around 11 P.M., taking sign-out from a colleague. I had not given much additional thought to the NRA's tweet since seeing it in the afternoon. I started to see new patients with my team.

Moments before midnight, a patient came with stroke-like symptoms. I sat in the CT scan control room with my team—a collection of emergency department residents, emergency nurses, and a neurology resident who had rushed to the emergency department after receiving the stroke alert page—while our patient was loaded on to the firm, slab-like gantry. While the CT scanner began to whir and the gantry began to move through the "donut of truth" I took a few quiet moments to click my phone back on to see what was going on in the world.

To my disgust, America had been struck with yet another mass shooting, this time in Thousand Oaks, California. The tragic irony was that it had happened fewer than twelve hours after the NRA's tweet. The irony was not lost on Dr. Kyle Fischer, an emergency physician at the University of Maryland. Fischer had sent me a message that said that the combination of the NRA's tweet and the recent tragedy in California had lit a fire under him.

Fischer is a typically level-headed Midwesterner, but his emotions were raw in that moment. He was tired of being told by special interests that he didn't have a right to speak up on a topic that he had expertise in, not only because of the emotional toll that losing a patient to gun violence takes on him, but because like many others—including Youkilis, Ranney, and myself—he had been trained in and understood the policy and politics behind the issues.

Fischer is both a physician and the policy director for the Health Alliance for Violence Intervention (HAVI). He was composing a written response to the NRA and requested my assistance. But as the CT scanner was powering down and I had to leave the dimly lit room to return to the harried pace of the night shift at one of Houston's two Level I trauma centers, I clicked my phone off, tucking it back into the left breast pocket of my navy blue scrubs. However, thoughts of a response reverberated incessantly in my mind.

After the long overnight shift, I arrived home on Thursday morning and sat down at the large, circular mahogany table in my dining room. I flipped open my laptop to see what Fischer had written overnight. I could see where he wanted to go with his thoughts. We had collaborated on gun policy in the past; Fischer had previously spoken at an Evidence-Based Health Policy Symposium I coordinated in Houston.

I took a spoonful of Raisin Bran Crunch, then furiously slapped at the keys on my MacBook Air—changing words, moving paragraphs, rephrasing sentences into what I thought would make for a convincing argument. As I looked up into the right upper corner of the Google document, I noted several other people adding pieces, recommending better language, and correcting mistakes. Nearly half a dozen physicians were simultaneously tweaking Fischer's letter, including Ranney.[7] A couple of hours later, my creative and physical energies exhausted, I closed my laptop.

I slept.

When I woke up, our retort to the NRA, incorporating the viral hashtag and exclaiming that "This Is Our Lane" was complete. Fischer, Ranney, and I published this op-ed piece in the *Houston Chronicle*:

> As physicians, we have sworn our lives to uphold a famous oath to obey the wise words of Hippocrates that implore us to "Cure sometimes, Treat often, Comfort always."
>
> Unfortunately, this is easier said than done amidst America's gun violence epidemic.
>
> It is not possible to cure every gunshot wound. Modern medical science has tremendously improved our ability to save lives. Emergency medical systems excel at rapidly treating and transporting victims; emergency physicians and trauma surgeons collaborate to stabilize patients, operate, and maximize the odds of survival. Yet still, for far too many people, once a bullet enters their body, cure may be impossible.
>
> For those who survive a gunshot, even those without disabling injuries, we must often treat both the visible and the invisible wounds that persist for a lifetime. Rehabilitation specialists help the injured restore their physical health, while psychiatrists and therapists piece together the mental well-being of those shattered in so many ways by firearm injuries. Post-traumatic stress disorder, something many incorrectly assume is a soldier's disease, haunts

patients for years after trauma. Simultaneously, we treat patients for decades after their initial injuries for complications like wound infections and bowel blockages. A rifle round tearing apart a body can lead to years of learning how to walk or talk again. Stitching up a wound in an operating room is not the end, but the beginning.

Too often, we are simply left to try to comfort the relatives of those who have died from their gunshot wounds. Too many of us have felt the weight of delivering bad news—the worst news—and only being able provide a shoulder to cry on, eventually leaving the newly bereaved alone in a sterile hospital "family room" to grieve. Anyone who has ever worked in a trauma bay can remember the visceral cry of a parent who has just been informed their son or daughter has died at the hand of a gun.

Last year, nearly 40,000 Americans died from firearm injuries. Tens of thousands more were injured but survived. We can only vaguely state tens of thousands because, if we're honest, we really do not know the exact number for that statistic. Plagued by decades of intentional policy decisions and under-funding, America lacks an accurate reporting system for non-fatal gunshot wounds.

When physicians do speak about the facts—and our own experiences—the National Rifle Association demands, to quote a recent tweet, that "someone should tell self-important anti-gun doctors to stay in their lane."

To be clear: We are not anti-gun. We are anti-bullet hole.

We see the impact of this epidemic in our daily lives, often leaving us with no real remedies beyond applying dressings, mending wounds. We are often forced to discharge our patients back to the same communities and situations that led to their initial injuries, newly scarred both inside and out.

As one of the leading causes of death for young people in America, gun violence must be addressed to prevent injuries and deaths. While we as doctors will continue to develop and refine medical science to save lives once a bullet strikes the flesh, it is our collective duty as a nation to prevent the bullet from striking our patients in the first place. We know that despite the efforts of physicians and nurses, once a trigger gets pulled, lives are changed forever.

Good research can make a difference. Medical research solved AIDS but physicians never took away sex. Medical research and public health interventions have dramatically reduced deaths and injury from car crashes but physicians never took away cars. Medical research can solve gun violence and firearm injury and physicians will not take away all guns.

We know how to prevent firearm-related deaths. Policies like universal background checks and allowing the temporary removal of firearms from individuals in crisis are proven to save lives. This election showed that the American people support these live-saving solutions—in fact, they're demanding them. As citizens and caregivers, we have a responsibility to speak up.

In response to the NRA's demand that we stay in our lane, we want to make one thing clear: **This is our lane**.[8]

Physicians, nurses, and many other health care workers seized on the #ThisIsOurLane hashtag over 30,000 times in the 72 hours following the Thousand Oaks shooting.[9] #ThisIsOurLane caught the attention of Americans across the country, and physicians around the world shared our disbelief that someone would assert that physicians didn't have a role in curbing the epidemic of gun violence in the United States. Never before had I seen the health care community speak with a strong and unified voice against the intimidations of the NRA. While some of our specialty organizations have had milquetoast statements about the dangers of firearms tucked away in their archives, physician organizations had rarely invested time and effort into advocating for the changes they wished to see. In fact, as we would come to appreciate in the following years, physician specialty organizations had donated substantial amounts of money to political candidates who had actively opposed efforts to end gun violence.[10]

But we had had enough.

We had had enough of the NRA's threats against the firearm injury prevention community and enough of the gun lobby's efforts to silence us. We were not about to stop speaking for those who had been unheard or those who could no longer speak for themselves. We figured that it was up to us to use our platforms on social media and in real life to amplify the voices of all those Americans whose lives had been cut short or irrevocably altered by the path of a bullet.

CHAPTER SEVEN

Rationally Irrational

I was never fond of guns growing up. Living in the suburbs of Washington, DC, whenever I heard of firearms it was in the context of someone being gunned down on the streets. In high school, television shows such as *Homicide: Life on the Street*, set in and filmed in nearby Baltimore, captivated me. The summer before I started college, my mother told me that Robbie had been added to the statistics of people killed by a bullet. Robbie, who was tall and lightly complected, raced across Winston-Salem that night, scanning the road as the nearly full moon cast shadows across his pointed nose and deep-set eyes. His gun, sitting there in the car, would soon fire that fateful bullet that would leave two children and four siblings without a father and a brother. Personally, I never felt the need for a gun—until one cold winter night in February 2014.

I was returning home from an emergency room shift. I had never felt unsafe in my sojourns through urban centers such as Washington, DC, Atlanta, and New York, cities I called home prior to moving to Houston. I parked my car in front of my house, unlocked the wrought-iron gate, and walked toward the front door in the darkness. The sun had already sunk below the winter sky.

The front door, painted a dark red, opened a little too easily.

Once inside, I crept into the foyer. Only a couple of steps inside the door, I noticed that all the lights were on, which was strange because my wife was supposed to be at work that evening and I was supposed to have arrived home first. With a hint of confusion, my eyes panned down and to the right. The bathroom door was ajar and drawers and cabinets had been flung open. Slowly, as my mind put the scene together, I realized what had happened.

What had happened was that someone had broken into my house!

Had I been a gun owner, I might have charged in recklessly, angrily, seeking to stop the bad guys with my gun. This is the precise situation in which the NRA proclaims that a good guy with a gun is supposed to intervene, to protect life and property and stop a criminal in their tracks. Instead, I backed out the door, unarmed and fearing that the thief might still be lurking inside with the means to harm me. Too nervous to even get in my own car, I slunk away from the house to a safe distance where I could see if anyone were to come or go from the front door but far enough away that they wouldn't notice me spying on my own residence. I called 911 in a panic, my pulse quickened. I provided the information they needed—a burglary was in process—and I waited.

Slowly, the adrenaline began to release its grip on my body. Warm blood, which had been shunted to my core as it would under any other fight-or-flight response, began returning to the periphery of my fingertips. My skin felt the intense cold air brush against me; my thin blue cotton scrubs offered almost no barrier to the weather.

While I waited anxiously for nearly 20 minutes for the Houston Police Department to arrive, my wife pulled up in her silver Volvo S60. I opened the passenger door and sat down on the black leather seats, eyes fixed on our eerily illuminated house. I flipped on the seat warmer.

About half an hour after I made the call, a black-and-white Houston Police Department squad car pulled up in front of the house with red and blue lights reflecting off the glass insert on the front door and living-room windows. I carefully stepped out of the Volvo and approached the police vehicle, making certain to keep my hands clearly visible to the officers. Wearing scrubs or not, as a Black man approaching the police responding to a burglary scene in the dead of night, I wasn't about to let them mistake me as someone who "fit the description."

The two police officers rolled down the window and listened to what I had to say. After hearing my story, one officer went around to the back of the house while the other one guarded the front door. Gun drawn, he ventured inside, shouting "Houston Police!" as he entered to clear the building.

A few minutes later, he assured me that the home was empty.

Still reeling from the thought that our personal sanctuary had been violated, we entered our home. As we walked through the foyer and entered the kitchen, I saw that a brown metallic file box had been pried open with an aluminum grilling fork. The papers had been ransacked but none were missing. To my left, shattered pieces of tempered glass from the French doors leading to the back porch lay on the hardwood floor, some embedded in a thick, orange circular carpet under the mahogany dining-room table. There I found our cat huddled for safety after becoming frightened from the unanticipated intrusion. She began to meow and purr when I picked her up. Thankfully, she hadn't run out into the cold black night.

Inside our home office, somehow, our computer remained. Of all the things to lose, that probably could have been the most devastating. It had memories of my entire life on it—writings and family photographs all existed in the memory of a computer instead of on paper and glossy prints. The drawers of the desk and the filing cabinet lay open.

I went upstairs, walking down the long, creaking hardwood corridor leading to the master bedroom. Inside the closet, the thief had found what they wanted—jewelry. Among the items taken were a Movado watch I had received from my wife for my birthday just a few weeks earlier. Two small cufflinks, emblazoned with Barack Obama's campaign logo and purchased from his campaign website during the summer of 2008, had also been taken. To this day, those cufflinks remain the one thing, aside from my piece of mind, that I wish I could have back.

When your home is broken into, it isn't the things that go missing that bother you, it is the loss of a sense of security the rattles you the most. After appraising our losses, we arranged for someone to drop by that night to replace the broken glass on the French doors. My wife thought that we needed something else to keep us safe in case the criminals attempted to return.

Growing up, I recall that my parents had always kept a blunt object, such as a wooden baseball bat, under the bed in case of emergencies. Carrying on that tradition, I have kept an old wooden bat, its grip long worn out and replaced by silver duct tape, under the bed. It dawned on me that cold February night that a weathered Louisville Slugger might not be adequate to repel any future armed attacks on our home. Perhaps having a gun wouldn't be so irrational after all.

I do not see eye to eye with the NRA or any of the other Second Amendment advocacy organizations now trying to take its place. But it should come as no surprise that like many Americans in general, even physicians choose to own and embrace firearms. Surveys differ, but the estimates of physician ownership of firearms range from 29 to 55%.[1] A 2021 study shows that even 43% of my emergency medicine colleagues own guns.[2]

Meanwhile, a large percentage of physicians who do not own firearms eschew guns because as children and adolescents, like me, they simply did not grow up in a culture fond of guns. Female physicians are less likely to own firearms than male physicians.[3] And firearm ownership among today's medical students tends to be lower than the general population, illustrating that the trend for firearm ownership is becoming less and less common among newer generations of doctors.[4]

A 2017 report from the Pew Research Center states that three in ten Americans own guns.[5] Two-thirds of gun owners report doing so for personal protection. One-third report hunting as a reason and nearly another third choose firearms for sports such as clay shooting or range shooting. A small portion, 13%, own guns as collectible keepsakes. Like most gun owners, I came into the possession of my first firearms for personal protection.

My wife went to Academy, a popular sporting-goods store in Texas, the day after our house was broken into and returned with a Maverick Model 88 12-gauge shotgun and a .40-caliber Smith and Wesson semiautomatic pistol. It surprised me how easily she was able to purchase them. No waiting period needed; just pass the instant background check and walk out with a weapon capable of destroying a life in a flash.

Until that day, I had never wanted to own a firearm. While some physicians might be opposed to keeping them at home because of the inherent risk of injury or death guns pose to occupants of the home (as Art Kellermann's research revealed), other physicians choose not to own or carry a weapon because of the color of their skin. Black and Brown physicians are not immune to the subtle—and often not-so-subtle—microaggressions and outright racist actions lodged against people of color in America. Growing up in a society that seems stacked against Black and Brown people and one in which law enforcement statistics reveal a disproportionate use of lethal force may be the main reason that physicians from minority backgrounds avoid carrying firearms. Police kill unarmed Black people at five times the rate that they kill unarmed white people.[6]

From 1999 to 2014, law enforcement officers across America killed 76 unarmed people of color.[7] On average, one unarmed person of color is killed by police every two months in the United States. And although police-involved shootings are rare in this country—just 611 fatalities in 2020—it is no wonder why some parents, me included, would never let our children play with toy guns, let alone get close to a real one.

Dr. Brian H. Williams is one such parent. A clean-shaven trauma surgeon, Williams experienced the intersection of race, guns, and medicine on a fateful summer night in Dallas in 2016 when he swapped trauma calls with one of his clinical partners.[8] He told me why he would not allow his daughter to play with a toy gun. He recalled Tamir Rice, a 12-year-old Black boy who was outside playing with a BB gun at a snowy park in Cleveland in 2014. Informed that a person was pointing a gun at people in the park, police hastily sped to the scene. In about ten minutes after the initial calls to 911, a dark police sedan drove onto the snowy lawn adjacent to a park bench where the boy had been sitting just moments earlier. In the flash of an eye, the passenger door to the police car burst open, shots were fired, and the boy fell to the ground. The next day, he was pronounced dead. After review of the incident by a grand jury, no charges were filed against the officer who gave Tamir Rice his fatal injuries.

Despite growing up in a military family, Williams, a Black man, never played with toy guns as a child. His parents wouldn't allow it. He attended the Air Force Academy, earning a degree in aeronautical engineering, and served actively in the air force for six years. But today he doesn't keep live firearms in his home.

Even among many affluent Black parents, there is too much realistic concern that someone might mistake a toy gun in the hands of a young Black boy or girl for a real weapon and either involve the police or, feeling threatened themselves, consider preemptive self-defense and take matters into their own hands.

In states with expansive Stand Your Ground laws, someone in fear for their safety has no duty to retreat when in public. Stand Your Ground legally permits people engaged in a potential conflict to escalate that conflict until they feel that deadly force is justified. As a result of these laws, some scientists estimate that 30 Americans die every month—roughly one American every day.[9,] In some places, especially southern states, Stand Your Ground laws are estimated to have resulted in an 8% increase in firearm homicides.[10]

The subconscious threatens the rational brain when you hear story after story of unarmed people of color killed by police, when Trayvon Martin can be stalked and killed yet the perpetrator can use Florida's Stand Your Ground law to escape prosecution. Or when a Minnesota police officer shoots a young Black man sitting in his own car after he had appropriately declared that he had a license to legally carry a firearm. It was the aftermath of this last shooting, one in which a concealed carry license contributed to a fatal outcome, that really hit home for me.

Philando Castile, a 32-year-old nutrition services supervisor at J.J. Hill Montessori Magnet School, was shot and killed during a traffic stop in the suburbs of St. Paul, Minnesota. I remember sitting in my office, taking a brief break from the hustle and bustle of the emergency department to scarf down a bite to eat, when the news flashed across my computer screen. The slaying of an innocent man, one who had gone through the procedures and was licensed to carry a firearm, shook me to my core. When I read that his four-year-old daughter had been seated in the back seat of the white Oldsmobile sedan and had been forced to witness her father's death—seven shots fired, five striking Castille, two ripping through his heart—I cried. All of this happened in just forty seconds from when the police officer began speaking with him to gunning him down. I wiped the tears from my face before returning to the doctors' station to continue that shift. That's one reason that I personally don't carry my firearm with me; Philando Castille's death scares me that another trigger-happy cop would be all too happy to end my life.

***

On the other hand, some physicians do carry their firearms when away from home. Dr. Stephanie Gordy is among them. A southern girl who grew up in the small town of LaGrange, Georgia, a little over an hour southwest of Atlanta, Gordy has retained a thick drawl. A tall blonde with piercing blue-green eyes and thin locks that wisp around in the wind, she gives off the air of a stereotypical southern belle. Her parents had kept a shotgun behind their door when Gordy was growing up and Gordy remembers her father using it to shoot the head of a snake. But she adopted a life that was opposed to violence and opposed to firearms. She was a self-described pacifist who left the Deep South after a lifetime in Georgia for a more progressive environment at Oregon Health & Science University, where she completed her surgical critical care fellowship.

Texas, where she later moved to practice, changed her views.

One day as she sat in her vehicle in a Houston hospital garage, leaving a voicemail for one of her surgical partners, a man wearing a hoodie approached her. The man walked right up to her driver door while she was largely unaware of her surroundings and knocked on the window, asking for a jump to restart his vehicle. At that exact moment, Gordy noticed that her driver's door was unlocked.

She wasn't sure if he intended to carjack her, to rob her, or to rape her—she instantaneously harbored suspicious feelings toward the man and decided that today was not the day to offer her help. The hairs on the back of her neck became erect, her skin moist with the sweat produced in the rush of the fight-or-flight response. She realized that she had nothing to fight back with except her fists—not even a scalpel. As the hooded man turned away, Gordy pushed a button on her door panel, locking herself inside the vehicle.

Realizing that in almost any situation, with the nearest hospital security guard over 50 yards away, she might be overwhelmed by a man's strength, Gordy felt powerless. Gordy appreciated the need to even the odds in case of a violent confrontation. That momentary feeling of fear and impotence set off inside of her mind a chain reaction that gradually began the process of breaking down her pacifism. After this incident, she bought her first firearm, a shotgun. Many Americans share these fears. Yet fear isn't an American phenomenon: guns are.

Following a second incident within six months after her move to Houston, when a strange car pulled into her secluded driveway and lingered too long, Gordy went ahead and obtained her Texas concealed carry license. Since then, she has gone on to become the stereotypical Texas gun owner, with multiple firearms in addition to her shotgun. She owns several handguns, a couple of shotguns, and an AR-15, which she described as a totally nonsensical purchase but one that was emotionally satisfying. Guns appeal to Gordy's sense of personal safety.

Following those two close encounters, Gordy discovered that one of her former romantic partners was stalking her. "Once you have a stalker you really never get the feeling of safety back, with or without a gun," she told me. "I think, with a gun it may just mitigate it a little more." The situation cemented her feelings that guns were a necessary part of her life.

Despite owning firearms and appreciating the pleasure she feels when shooting her ArmaLite rifle, as a trauma surgeon, Gordy recognizes the catastrophic damage AR-15s and similarly designed weapons can inflict on the human body.

"It's pretty terrifying," she told me, describing the amount of damage a weapon like an AR-15 inflicted on one of her patients, a young woman who had a gaping hole in her back and flank. On the operating room table, Gordy could put her whole hand through the wound and touch the leather-like upholstery of the operating table. The arc of her life, from the pacifist southerner opposed to guns to a Texas trauma surgeon sporting a semi-automatic rifle with a concealed carry license, is one of great transition and evolution. Having moved from far left to moderate in her political views, Gordy, like most gun owners, doesn't think that the gun itself is the problem; violence, on the other hand, is. She shares that view with the NRA.

Viewing gun violence from the lens of public health, Gordy views certain societal ills—poverty, crime, gangs, unstable social situations, lack of education—as the birthplace of violence.

To a degree, she is correct. As I've written earlier, firearms are merely vectors for violence. Gordy disagrees with the NRA's approach, calling them overly polarizing.

As a gun owner and a physician, Gordy, respects researchers such as Arthur Kellermann and Megan Ranney as well as survivors of gun violence and families of victims. For me, as someone who has devoted himself to advocacy to save lives, the science is key, but so too are the opinions of gun owners. To successfully grapple with endemic gun violence that continues to propel person after person into our emergency rooms, trauma bays, operating rooms, and morgues , we need more than just stories.

The plural of anecdote isn't data.

We need both narrative and evidence if we are ever to stop this plague of gun violence infecting our country.

CHAPTER EIGHT

A Well-Regulated Militia

D r. Edwin Leap peered out of the small plexiglass window of the Life Flight helicopter as the aircraft swiftly descended to the scene, his eyes straining to make out the contours of the victim, a man who had tried to take his own life by pointing a .45-caliber pistol to the side of his head and pulling the trigger. The helicopter touched down on a flat portion of the field where bystanders had found the man. Blood, vomit, and brain splatter stained the grass as blue and red lights flashed noiselessly from the fire truck and ambulance assembled at the scene. The deafening whir of the helicopter's rotors drowned out everything else as Leap jumped past the metallic beast whose engines continued to growl, ready to rev back up if the physician could stabilize the patient and return him to the helicopter. That was Leap's task, to ensure that the patient survived long enough to make it on board.

Leap hollered orders at the paramedics standing by. He knelt down, feeling the mud seep through his flight suit, and took a look at the man. He wasn't breathing. Pushing away the hands of the paramedic who was pushing oxygen into the man's lungs through an Ambu bag, Leap wiggled his jaw, found it stiff, and requested medications to paralyze the man. Already having drawn up the medications in anticipation of the need to secure the airway prior to flight, a flight nurse pushed the clear fluid through an intravenous line and within seconds, the man ceased breathing. That was Leap's opportunity.

Looking into the man's throat with a curved steel blade designed to press the tongue out of the way and peer down to the vocal cords, Leap held out his hand and with his rapid southern twang, asked for an endotracheal tube, a long piece of curved plastic that would deliver oxygen to the lungs. After the flight nurse slipped the tube into Leap's steady hand, he advanced it past the vocal cords into the patient's airway and secured the tube. Moments later, after confirming that both lungs had inflated equally, the pair loaded the man onto the helicopter, which swiftly lifted off from the scene to rush to the trauma center.

Decades later, Leap, a middle-aged fair-skinned man from rural South Carolina, sits at home, stroking a graying goatee and looking through the emergency medicine magazine for jobs. In his extensive career as an emergency physician, he has worked in environments such as urgent care centers, in small and mid-sized community hospitals, and in critical-access hospitals in rural areas like where he grew up and now lives. The memory of the man lying in the muck after having tried to take his own life remains fresh in Leap's mind.

Leap has worked as what we call in our business a locum tenens physician, going from hospital to hospital filling holes in schedules and earning a good amount of money doing so. Never fully invested in one place, he and the other locum physicians like him are vital resources at each place where they choose to spend their time. But for the time being, staying away from the front lines of coronavirus wasn't such a bad thing, Leap suggested, for a physician like him who, based on his age, fell into the higher-risk demographic.

Finding no opportunities in the advertisements to suit his tastes that day, Leap fiddled with his guns instead. He had grown up around guns. "In dad's dresser, in the closet, in the neighbor's truck. It's what I knew," he says. His ownership of firearms began as early as childhood. In college, Leap spent time in the Reserve Officer Training Corps. After becoming a practicing emergency physician, he spent several weeks as a flight surgeon. He muses that even in the parking lots of the rural hospitals where he has worked, one out of every three vehicles would house a firearm.

Sitting on the porch of his rural South Carolina home that sits on a 50-acre parcel of land, Leap has ample time to reflect on the cases he has witnessed over the decades of his clinical practice. And although he has witnessed some terrible things, some of which were brought on by guns, it is a stabbing, one in which a woman was knifed twelve times in the back, that haunts him the most.

That incident occurred in Indianapolis, when Leap attended medical school at a place that was once called Methodist Hospital of Indiana, now just IU Health Methodist Hospital. Back at home in South Carolina, as an independently practicing emergency physician, Leap remembers the emergency thoracotomy, the proverbial "cracking of the chest" when a patient of penetrating trauma, afflicted by a knife or a bullet wound, loses their pulses and the doctors must reach inside the body, place a clamp across the aorta—the huge blood vessel coming directly off the heart—and see if there are any salvageable injuries that can be fixed. It's not an easy task for the uninitiated.

One study of cases in which the emergency physician or trauma surgeon must cut an opening from the breastbone, under the nipple, and across the chest toward the armpit found that fewer than 8% of patients who undergo an emergency department thoracotomy survived.[1] In cases where the patient ultimately succumbs to their injuries, often a penetrating wound to the heart or the major blood vessels, the physician standing on that side of the stretcher gets covered in blood as he or she scoops out several pints of congealed blood, which has the look and feel and sound of canned cranberry sauce as it plops to the floor of the trauma bay.

Leap has performed three of these desperate lifesaving procedures in his career, all for stab wounds to the heart. Even if only one of the three patients on which Leap performed a thoracotomy survived their injuries, it would have been considered a miracle. Certainly it would have been beating the odds. That woman's face, the one stabbed a dozen times, used to invade Leap's thoughts; her face kept him up at night. The victims of gun violence never do.

But he does vividly remember one case.

A nurse, not anyone that Leap had worked with in the past, depressed over the fact that his girlfriend had broken up with him, tried to take his own life. Distraught, he thought the only way to cure the pain was to point a shotgun at himself and attempt suicide. The pellets from the shotgun penetrated the abdomen, striking his liver and shattering it into pieces. The liver is one of two major organs that when injured severely enough in a car wreck or from a stabbing or gunshot wound can bleed what seems like indefinitely (the other is the spleen). As the saying goes, all bleeding stops eventually. In the case of a fatal trauma, the bleeding stops when the patient runs out of blood.

The shotgun left pellets on top of pellets, according to Leap, essentially liquefying the man's liver with every breath he took. Bits and chunks of brown liver bubbled from the open wound as the man's diaphragm oscillated up and down. Leap remembers the surgeon on call that day shaking his head in dismay at an overwhelming and unsalvageable situation.

Unlike the urban interpersonal violence I and Stephanie Gordy have witnessed in one of Houston's trauma centers, Leap's experience with gun violence is the type responsible for most firearm deaths. According to the CDC, suicide by firearm killed 24,292 Americans in 2020.[2] Historically, firearm suicides are nearly double the number of firearm homicides and they dwarf the numbers of unintentional deaths caused by children stumbling across a loaded weapon. As a top ten cause of death in America, suicide should concern us all, whether we have experienced mental health issues firsthand or not. The impulsivity of the act can result in someone taking their life in less than an hour from the initial thought if the fatal means are accessible.

***

A few months before the NRA attacked the medical profession with its poorly thought out tweet, Leap wrote an opinion piece from the perspective of a gun owner and a physician. It was an attempt to create a bridge between those who want unfettered access to any firearm without regard to their inherit dangers and those who seek to ban guns outright without regard for Americans' interests in owning them.[3] He was specifically addressing the topic of owning the AR-15, a common weapon retrieved in recent mass shootings that often turn out to be horrific examples of murder-suicides. As a physician, a gun owner, and a parent, Leap's thoughts on firearms are understandable to almost any reasonable American. However, the unreasonable viewed his ideas about assault weapons and who should possess them as offensive.

Leap recommended that anyone who wanted to own such weapons follow the same process that South Carolina uses to vet people for concealed carry permits: fingerprinting, a background check, and a four-hour class to discuss the safety and legal ramifications of shooting a firearm and to assess for competence. Leap passed these tests himself to obtain a South Carolina concealed carry permit. Following this, Leap recommends a two-month waiting period. After that, the state would issue a card that would allow the holder to buy a gun whenever he or she presented it to a federal firearms licensed dealer. There wouldn't be a limitation on the number of guns he or she could obtain because that individual had already been vetted as being safe.

For Leap, specific weapons such as the ArmaLite AR-15 and similar sporting rifles should be restricted to individuals over the age of 21. As we will learn later in this book, the data supports restrictions on firearms for people under the age of 21. Leap believes there should be an exception to a potential age restriction on ownership of assault weapons, which are designed to function similarly to the M-16, their military cousin. "If you can go to war," Leap said of young people who have been screened by the military and passed weapons training, "you can be trusted."

I believe Leap's ideas are reasonable. However, some Second Amendment zealots assume that his ideas are the first step on the road to serfdom and tyranny. Others on the opposite end of the spectrum feel like the United States should simply ban assault weapons outright.

For a decade, from 1994 to 2004, America did that. There was a ban on the manufacture and sale of assault weapon–style rifles in the United States. The law was passed during the Clinton administration along with other gun regulations such as the Brady background check. The assault weapons ban was even supported by former presidents Gerald Ford, Ronald Reagan, and Jimmy Carter, who cited the statistic that "although assault weapons account for less than 1% of the guns in circulation, they account for nearly 10% of the guns traced to crime."[4]

It has been two decades since this experiment ended. What have we learned?

Assault weapons such as the ArmaLite AR-15 are formally called center-fire semiautomatic rifles and typically resemble the US military M-16 in that they have pistol grips and detachable magazines. However, unlike military weapons, civilian assault weapons are limited to semiautomatic fire and cannot perform selective fire—that is, they do not allow the operator to choose between fully automatic, semiautomatic, or burst modes of fire. Today, a ban on assault weapons has become one of the more controversial gun control policies debated in the United States. The assault weapons ban lasted ten years, expired, and was not renewed. These types of sporting rifles can lay down a series of rapid and powerful gunfire in a matter of seconds. The perpetrators in many of the mass shootings in our nation's recent history have made use of sporting rifles like this for precisely that reason—they efficiently kill and maim as many as possible in as short a time frame as possible especially when coupled to magazines that can carry a large amount of ammunition.

In 1996, following a shooting in the Australian town of Port Arthur that killed 35 people, that country's prime minister, John Howard, the leader of a center-right political coalition, led a movement to ban semiautomatic and automatic weapons. Australia's firearms ban included a national gun buyback in which

650,000 guns were removed from circulation. Since taking those actions, which also included implementing waiting periods before purchase, a firearm registry, and strict licensing rules, Australia has not seen another mass shooting, yet Australians still own 3.5 million *registered* firearms.[5]

Americans who support gun safety often point to the US Violent Crime Control and Law Enforcement Act of 1994 (colloquially known as the assault weapons ban) as evidence that mass shootings could decline in the United States if a ban was resumed. Although seven states and the District of Columbia have banned assault weapons, the empirical data provided by the RAND Corporation's *The Science of Gun Policy*, the analysis the National Rifle Association used to claim that physicians were stepping outside their lane, suggests that there is insufficient evidence for these claims.[6]

You might not believe what I just wrote.

I'll admit it; the gun lobby is correct here. The evidence analyzed by *The Science of Gun Policy* does not currently indicate that a ban on assault weapons will save people's lives. But that's the premise upon which *this* book is based—whether certain firearm policies will improve morbidity and mortality in America—and it's the metric upon which I formulate my personal beliefs about gun policy.

I have faith in evidence-based health policy. From here on out in this book, that's what we will do, explore the data to see what firearms policies the evidence says can help save American lives.

Policy Prescription: A Ban on Assault Weapons Might Not Save Lives

Even though assault weapons have commonly been used in mass shootings like Sandy Hook and in the mass killings of law enforcement officers, the data are inconclusive about the effect of an assault weapons ban on mass shootings. The data similarly are unable to prove that the assault weapons ban correlated to a reduction in total homicides and firearm homicides. Although the lay public and clinicians alike can recognize the destructive power of firearms such as the AR-15, the science has yet to bear out the benefits of the proposed solution.

According to the science, the only thing that banning assault weapons would accomplish is a transient increase in the price of these types of firearms. Whether or not these price increases would put these guns out of reach for those who would like to do harm to the greatest number of people remains unknown.

A chilling story by John Woodrow Cox in his book *Children under Fire* shows that cost isn't always the barrier for would-be killers. It wasn't the barrier for the teenager who murdered a young boy at Townville Elementary in South Carolina. The young man had intended to use his father's Ruger Mini-14 to invoke massive bloodshed.[7] He assumed that the rifle was locked in a gun safe; that was the only thing that kept the Townville shooting from becoming a household name like Sandy Hook. In fact, the Mini-14 was just out of view, unlocked and accessible.

Avid gun owners such as Leap have ideas about how to keep the AR-15 and similar weapons like the Mini-14 legal, the killing of innocent civilians rare, and the use of these sporting rifles by law-abiding gun owners safe. Like Leap, I agree that a ban on assault weapons is not as important as other policies that would focus on the individual holding the weapon rather than the weapon being held.

The NRA is fond of saying that "guns don't kill people; people kill people." If that's truly the case and we don't need to regulate the machinery that arms the militia, shouldn't we regulate the people who constitute the militia? I have wondered why the NRA opposes conducting a background check on every person who wants to own a gun, since its members believe that it is people and not guns that are responsible for over 45,000 firearm-related deaths every year. Instead, the NRA remains complacent about the fact that in America, 22% of gun purchases evade the background check process.[8]

- Banning assault weapons will lead to a transient increase in the price of these types of firearms, but it might not save lives.

CHAPTER NINE

An Ounce of Prevention

A 70-year-old man wearing a brand-new dark-blue suit with a French-cuffed white shirt walked out of the Washington Hilton Hotel on an overcast day, waving his right hand to onlookers. He was flanked by a man in a beige trench coat on the right. One of his aides, about half a foot shorter and thirty years his junior, strolled a step behind him on his left.

Suddenly, six shots in 1.7 seconds.

A bullet ricocheted and punched a small opening below the older man's left armpit. His security detail shoved him forcefully into a waiting car that sped off toward the White House.

President Reagan had been shot.

The trauma surgeon who happened to be on call that day at George Washington University Hospital, the institution where I would eventually train in emergency medicine, was Dr. Joseph Giordano. He walked down to see his patient, the president of the United States, as the trauma team was already evaluating him.[1] Reagan lay stark naked on the gurney. No recognizable sounds were coming from his left lung.[2] In fact, the president's lung had collapsed under the pressure of the continuous bleeding inside his chest. The team quickly inserted a chest tube, but the bleeding continued. "The would-be assassin must have struck an artery," Dr. Giordano thought, processing the possible injuries the president might have sustained. Reagan would need an operation to fix a pulmonary artery injury.

Before going under anesthesia, Reagan reportedly said to the doctors, "I hope you all are Republicans."

After a brief chuckle, the surgeon, a liberal Democrat, replied. "Today, Mr. President, we are all Republicans."

Back at the crime scene, Jim Brady, who had been struck in the head by the first bullet and who had fallen face first onto the concrete, was bleeding from the left side of his face. He had sustained the most devastating injuries of the four people who were shot that day. Rumors quickly swirled around DC that he had been killed. Instead, Brady lay in a pool of warm blood and cold rain, partially paralyzed. The firearm injury he sustained that day left him with slurred speech and would require that he use a wheelchair for the remainder of his life.

Brady, Reagan's press secretary, would later lead the advocacy effort for stricter gun control laws with his wife, Sarah. Success would not arrive until two presidential administrations later when their efforts were finally rewarded by the passage of the Brady Handgun Violence Prevention Act in 1993—one of the critical pieces of gun legislation signed by President Bill Clinton.

The Brady Act established the background check process that Americans today go through to buy a gun. Pushed forward by Brady, a lifelong Republican, and signed by President Clinton, a Democrat, background checks should not be contrived as either a blue state or a red state issue. Background checks on every gun purchase, which are common in many other nations that permit their citizens to own guns, are a controversial issue in America. But in a country where the disease of violence is amplified by the easy accessibility of guns, wouldn't requiring a background check for every gun purchase seem prudent? Most Americans think so. In 2017, a Gallup poll showed that 96% of all Americans favor requiring background checks on *all* gun purchases.[3]

The Brady Act, which passed against the opposition of the NRA, established a national system to screen potential firearms buyers and to keep weapons out of the hands of individuals deemed too dangerous to exercise their individual constitutional right to bear arms. The National Instant Criminal Background Check System (NICS) has performed over 333 million checks on potential gun buyers since 1998.[4] It has denied nearly 1.7 million firearms purchases to individuals who fit one or more of the following conditions: people who have been convicted of a crime punishable by imprisonment for more than one year (i.e., felonies); fugitives from justice; people who are addicted to controlled substances; people who have been deemed mentally defective or who have been committed to a mental institution; undocumented people who are unlawfully present in the United States; individuals dishonorably discharged from the armed forces; individuals who have renounced US citizenship; people subject to a court restraining order for harassing, stalking, or threatening an intimate partner or the child of an intimate partner; and people convicted of misdemeanor domestic violence.

But the Brady background check process does not apply to every firearm transaction. Person-to-person private sales do not require the seller to perform a background check or even to record the sale. This gap in the law creates a loophole that allows firearms to be diverted from law-abiding Americans to those with more nefarious intent.

If we go back to the public health analogy, background checks represent a type of primary prevention. Primary prevention, in the context of disease transmission, means preventing disease before it can occur.

When I think about guns, I think about small insects that feed off humans—mosquitos. These tiny murderous beasts kill twice as many people as humans do. In the public health analogy, mosquitos are no different than a .22-caliber handgun or a sporting rifle. They are the deadliest animal on the planet—even deadlier than gun-toting humans.

These biting insects are a mild annoyance for some; we notice the bite and then are left to scratch. However, some of these bugs serve as vectors for deadly diseases such as malaria, dengue, Zika virus, and West Nile virus. Occasionally, although it seems really difficult to imagine, these tiny creatures serve a valuable purpose in our world. For instance, if you like orchids—and if you like vanilla-flavored anything then you really like orchids—you rely on mosquitoes to pollinate the flowers of those elongated, beautiful flowering plants with their tiny tongues.[5]

If you don't really care for orchids, you might be wondering, Why don't we just wipe these critters off the face of the planet? In one fell swoop, we'd save millions of lives and eradicate dozens of mosquito-borne diseases. But as much as we hate them, we probably need them (and not just for vanilla ice cream). Eradicating mosquitoes could potentially be detrimental to the ecosystem in ways we don't yet understand.

You might think that eliminating every gun in America would stop every instance of gun violence. You wouldn't be wrong. You can't have gun deaths without guns.

That is exactly how some people think about guns in the United States—assuming that every firearm is a deadly nuisance that needs to be eliminated. Others might argue that we don't need to eliminate every gun, just certain ones like the ArmaLite AR-15. But as I mentioned in the last chapter, there isn't clear evidence that banning assault weapons will save lives on a large scale.

Just as we don't need to eliminate every gun in this country to reduce gun deaths, we probably don't need to eliminate every mosquito on earth to stop the spread of malaria and the other deadly diseases they carry. Of the nearly 4,000 mosquito species in the world, only a few hundred serve as vectors for disease. Perhaps we could isolate our rage against a specific mosquito such as *Aedes aegypti*, the vector for malaria, dengue, and Zika.

I've spoken about gun violence in front of many audiences. One day after I gave a talk about the public health approach to gun violence prevention to a group of doctors, a tall, older physician from Alaska approached me to discuss what he called "gun control." He impressed on me his need to always keep a firearm nearby and not because of gangs or criminals. One day a far more ferocious threat stood between his front door and his truck. Perched an arm's length away was a massive brown bear. Its fur was grizzled and standing up at the nape of its neck, and he thought the bear would attack. Instead, it turned and fled. But instances like this are why he always keeps a firearm on his person whenever he drives across rural Alaska.

Another physician from New York told me that no American needed AR-15s. A former military member who had witnessed the killing power of the assault rifles capable of fully automatic fire upon which the AR-15 is modeled, he divulged his position regarding "weapons of war" in the hands of civilians, explaining that since its assault weapons ban in 1996, Australia has not experienced mass shootings like the carnage unleashed in America at a rate of greater than one mass shooting per day.[6] In America in 2020, there were 610 mass shootings—defined as episodes where at least four people are shot in one incident—nearly two per day.[7] Subsequent years have eclipsed that pace of mass violence.

These two physicians, united by their profession but divided by their take on guns, exemplify why the solution to our gun violence epidemic isn't so simple. Much like dealing with mosquito-borne disease, Americans must take a multifaceted public health approach to address the firearm-borne disease. How do we address the disease agent itself? How do we address means reduction via the gun vector? How do we prevent the recurrence of disease?

Violence—bred by hate, bigotry, misogyny, depression, suicidality—that's the disease we are fighting. Addressing these issues also includes focusing on the means by which this disease is transmitted from one human reservoir to the next human host.

Personally, I do not think that it is rational or necessary to eliminate every gun in the United States. It is certainly irrational to not do *something* about guns. Although millions of Americans enjoy safely shooting firearms for sport and hunting or for protection, over 120,000 Americans are killed or injured by firearms every year.[8]

Perhaps it is possible to ban and buy back all AR-15s, as Australia did. But I doubt that America would follow this course. With persistent fearmongering from the NRA and the Second Amendment protecting the individual's right to bear arms, I do not believe that will ever be a valid option. However, we should find palatable ways to regulate and control the use of these tools similar to how we dump standing water and spray insecticides in our efforts to control mosquitos and prevent the spread of the diseases they spread.

The first clause of the Second Amendment, which bestows on every American the right to bear arms, also implies that that right should be *well-regulated*. There can be no doubt that the threat to mortality with a weapon as powerful as a semiautomatic center-fire rifle is much greater than that from a small-caliber pistol. Yet odds are that vastly more people will be killed by handguns in the United States than by AR-15s. For every death from a rifle like an AR-15, handguns cause nineteen other deaths.

How we address these deaths requires a multipronged approach. Some aspects need to be focused on primary prevention. The Brady Act is a perfect example of this stratagem. In the case of gun violence, background checks exist as a form of vector control, keeping guns—the mechanism by which anger, hate, and suicidality are transmitted—out of the hands of the wrong people, thereby preventing violent injuries and death. Background checks represent one way to cut down on the transmission of hostilities between two people—or the inflicting of personal harm—via a bullet.

Over one out of every five firearms transactions occur without such vetting.[9] Why haven't we improved and expanded the background check process to make it more difficult for firearms to go from the hands of honorable people into the hands of those who wish to harm others?

The Brady background check has prevented nearly 1.7 million transactions, a rejection rate of approximately 0.5% for gun sales or permits to prohibited buyers. But what if a buyer tries to skirt the background check process? If we were to extrapolate the number of rejected background checks onto the number of transactions that occur outside the official NICS background check system, we would find that there might already be over 400,000 guns floating around this country in the hands of people who should not have them.

CHAPTER TEN

A Pound of Cure

Joe Sakran, a gun violence prevention advocate, speaks out on the topic of background checks with a sanguine and personal tone in his voice. One day in the fall of 1994, Sakran had just finished an SAT prep class. A friend was waiting for him at home to take him to the first game of the high school football season. He was in such a rush that he muttered only "I gotta go!" to his parents as he left the house.

"Afterwards, hanging out with friends at a nearby house," he explained, "a fight broke out that we had nothing to do with, and a guy pulled out a gun and started firing into the crowd." The gunman, a teenage El Salvadorian immigrant, indiscriminately fired into the crowd of young men and women. One of the bullets struck Sakran. Its energy, now transferred to the body of the young, college-bound teenager, ruptured his windpipe, damaged his carotid artery, and paralyzed one of his vocal cords.

"God was like, you know, watching over me," he reflected, thinking about how he could have bled to death that evening. Or he could have been completely paralyzed from a bullet shattering his spinal cord. Instead, Sakran was scooped up by an ambulance crew, bloodied and barely breathing.

Paramedics unloaded Sakran into the oversized trauma bay of Inova Fairfax Hospital. A nurse, a young resident physician, and Dr. Bob Ahmed, the general surgeon coordinating trauma care that day, attended to Sakran's injury. Seeing the blood pouring from his neck and hearing the air bubbling from his broken windpipe, Ahmed knew there was no time to waste. Sakran was rushed into emergency surgery to repair his blood vessels and his burst windpipe. Over the next month, Sakran would undergo multiple surgeries from two additional surgeons—Dr. Dipankar Mukherjee, a vascular surgeon from India who repaired Sakran's severed blood vessels, and Dr. Tim McBride, a pediatric otolaryngologist, who restored his voice. The bullet that ripped his trachea apart altered Sakran's voice for good. His raspy intonation has become the memorable trademark of a man who suffered a horrific personal trauma at a young age. Sakran spent the next six months with a plastic tube sticking out of his neck so he could breathe.

In the emergency department, I usually don't see people with tracheostomy tubes other than those who are stuck on ventilators for extended periods of time. I remember hearing Christopher Reeve, the actor who portrayed Superman in the late 1970s and early 1980s, speak at my medical school following the life-altering equestrian injury in which he broke his neck.

I've seen countless patients suffer cancer of the voice box, or larynx, and have to undergo a laryngectomy. This cure for their cancer eliminates their voice box so that only an opening from their lungs to the front of the neck remains and they breathe through a tracheostomy tube. For a teenage boy like Sakran, that could have been emotionally devastating.

Nevertheless, Sakran persisted. After graduating from high school and attending college at George Mason University in northern Virginia, he moved across the world to study medicine in Israel. The boy with the altered voice returned home a doctor and became a trainee at the hands of the same surgeons who had saved his life.

Sakran remembered operating with Mukherjee—the surgeon who had repaired his own blood vessels—on a delicate vascular procedure. Sakran's hands were shaking because he was nervous and he moved his hand abruptly. Beads of sweat pooled under the blue surgical cap covering his head. "Joe, did you take your Parkinson's meds?" Mukherjee joked, his eyes fixed on the ropey, pulsating blood vessel before them as a surgical mask hid a wry smile.

A moment of levity in what was otherwise a nerve-wracking experience. How would you feel standing across a narrow black table, clothed in blue sterile surgical garb, with your hands deep inside someone's body repairing a ruptured aorta with the same man who had once saved your own life a few years earlier? Practicing in his hometown and training to give others a second chance was one of the greatest experiences of his life, Sakran said. But like many people in medicine, especially those fighting against the pain caused by gun violence, saving one life just wasn't enough. Sakran decided he would use his voice—as well as his surgical skills—to advocate for gun violence victims.

By the time I sat with Sakran in Baltimore—where he is an associate professor of surgery at The Johns Hopkins Hospital— 25 years had passed since he was shot and he had published more than a dozen articles on gun violence. One of his studies of gun violence won an award for its calculation of the cost of gun violence to America: $2.8 billion each year.[1] His advocacy landed him on the board of the Brady Campaign to Prevent Gun Violence and the Brady Center, gun violence prevention organizations that had been renamed in honor of President Reagan's press secretary. Sakran had just finished speaking at the National Leadership Conference for Doctors for America, an organization whose board I had recently joined, when we sat in the back of a large hall to talk.

In a sky-blue two-button blazer over a white collared dress shirt, Sakran sat across from me as he discussed the Haddon Matrix, a widely used framework in the field of injury prevention. Developed by William Haddon in 1970, the matrix looks at various factors related to a person's injury or death, such as their environment, their personal attributes, and the thing that killed or injured them. In his landmark article, Haddon argued that injuries are a part of being human, have always been endemic to human society, and are therefore subject to the same epidemiological analogies public health providers use when they approach traditional diseases. Haddon, interestingly, erased the arbitrary line between acute injury and chronic disease by examining certain conditions from the perspective of the span of time.[2]

Consider the fate of a 26-year-old jogger who happens to be running past an old oak tree when one of its boughs, damaged by a recent storm, breaks away from the tree and lands on him. The immediate weight of the massive branch fractures his spine and paralyzes him. Most people would think of this acute event as an *injury*.

Now imagine a different type of injury, one that occurs incrementally over years and years of wear and tear on the spine. Eventually, the little openings between the vertebrae, known as the spinal foramen, narrow and scar, leading to a disease called spinal stenosis, sometimes described as arthritis of the spine. The person with spinal stenosis will feel sciatica and experience numbness and shooting pains down the back of their legs and even paralysis in extreme cases.

In the case of oak branch versus the jogger, we consider the falling-branch event a traumatic injury but think of the stenosed spine as a chronic disease—one of the joys of aging. Yet both are secondary to compression of the spine and both eventually damage the spinal cord and nerves. The difference between the two is just a matter of time. In Haddon's mind and in the mind of injury prevention professionals such as Sakran, the two processes are merely different parts of the same spectrum.

The Haddon Matrix, Sakran explained to me, applies the same concepts that epidemiologists and disease detectives use—concepts such as agents of disease, vehicles and vectors, and the host's susceptibility—to injurious agents. Haddon converted the three phases of prevention—primary, secondary, and tertiary—into one axis of his matrix for injury prevention. The other axis of the matrix covers the human, vector, and environmental factors that influence each component of an injury.

From the Haddon Matrix comes strategies the injury prevention specialist can use to approach these problems. These tactics ultimately reduce the impact of disease on people. Would any of these strategies have prevented Sakran from getting shot in the neck when he was a teenager? To address that question, it makes sense to look at the Haddon Matrix specifically from the perspective of interpersonal violence.

Our focus is on the agent of injury (violence), not necessarily the vector (the gun). What can we do in the first phase, the time before the actual traumatic event occurs, to reduce the risk of being shot? One potential strategy for reducing firearm injuries and deaths includes making sure that only law-abiding

TABLE 10.1. The Haddon Matrix applied to personal violence

	Host	Agent	Environment
Pre-Event	Limit walking alone at night in high-crime areas	Universal background checks on all firearms sales Keep firearms at home unloaded and locked	Add streetlights to enhance lighting
Event	Avoid escalating conflicts	Enforce firearm restrictions on people with felony convictions	Identify and clean up illicit drug trade
Post-Event	"STOP THE BLEED®"* courses for members of the community	Trace firearms involved in a shooting to determine liability	Invest in trauma centers and violence intervention programs

*STOP THE BLEED® is a program of the American College of Surgeons that has trained over 3 million people worldwide to recognize life threatening bleeding and teaches three methods of hemorrhage control to first responders. Visit https://www.stopthebleed.org to learn more.

Source: Adapted from Richmond TS, Forman M. Firearm violence: a global priority for nursing science. *J Nurs Scholarsh*. 2019 May;51(3):229–240.

citizens have access to firearms. Conducting instantaneous background checks with complete and reliable data on every gun sale must therefore be a priority. This is the essence of primary prevention.

But once guns are in the home, we must turn to secondary prevention efforts to prevent injury. Secondary prevention is akin to cancer screening. It tries to detect disease in its early stages and treat it before symptoms appear. You can think of secondary prevention as keeping guns safe inside the home, for example: making sure they are stored unloaded and locked in cabinets separate from ammunition.

Sakran, as a trauma surgeon, gun violence survivor, and advocate for gun safety, spends much of his time thinking about primary and secondary prevention strategies. The Brady Campaign to Prevent Gun Violence works to improve and expand instant background checks before an individual can purchase a firearm and to ensure that guns are stored safely to prevent unintentional injuries, something advocates call family fire.

Few physicians can empathize with victims of firearm injury like Sakran can. In the late 2000s, he spent every third night running the surgical ICU as a senior surgical resident at Inova Fairfax Hospital. Sakran is a bulky guy, and his faint, hoarse voice counters his outward appearance. He isn't the stereotypical angry, loud-mouthed, scalpel-throwing, overconfident surgeon. Even under the greatest stress, Sakran was nice to be around. I should know; he trained me.

As part of my residency training at George Washington University, I spent two months at Inova Fairfax Hospital embedded with the surgical critical care service, the trauma team where Sakran was the senior resident on service. He was one of the many surgeons who taught me how to care for the trauma victim, whether their calamity was the result of a fall, a car crash, a stabbing, or, occasionally, a bullet. During my two months in the trauma ICU, I learned that Sakran was gentle toward his team, respectful to his supervisors, and, most important, a passionate advocate for his patients. One day I noticed the scar on his neck. Before the end of my rotation with the trauma team at Inova Fairfax, Sakran told me how he had earned that scratchy voice. Sakran will tell his story to anyone who will listen, describing the bullet that changed his life, the one that he has kept on display on the dresser in his home for years.

Policy Prescription: Universal Background Checks Will Save Lives

The Gun Control Act of 1968, passed in the wake of the assassinations of President John F. Kennedy, Rev. Martin Luther King Jr., and Robert Kennedy, put in place an honor system in which potential gun buyers had to attest that they were legally permitted to own a gun. The act forbade criminals, felons, and people with serious mental health issues from purchasing firearms and prohibited sales by mail order, the method by which Lee Harvey Oswald obtained the rifle he used to kill President Kennedy.[3]

Following the attempt to assassinate President Reagan and the serious injuries sustained by his press secretary, James Brady, momentum once again built around creating a more robust background check process. Although early attempts at passage stalled when President George H. W. Bush, an NRA Life Member, refused to sign the Brady Bill in 1992, the act eventually passed in 1993 under the Clinton administration. It created a system in which federal firearms licensed dealers could cross-reference a database against potential purchasers and limit transfers of deadly weapons to people who should not own guns.[4]

The Brady Act created the FBI's National Instant Criminal Background Check System (NICS) and banned several classes of people from purchasing firearms from federal firearms licensed dealers. These included people convicted of felonies with prison terms that lasted longer than one year; fugitives from justice; people addicted to controlled substances; people committed to mental institutions; undocumented immigrants; people dishonorably discharged from the armed forces; people who have renounced US citizenship; people subject to a court restraining order for harassing, stalking, or threatening an intimate partner or the child of an intimate partner; and anyone convicted of misdemeanor domestic violence.

Out of the 333 million transactions processed through the NICS background check system since its inception in 1998, 1.7 million have been denied, according to a 2019 Justice Department report.[5] Of these potential transactions, nearly half were rejected because the attempted purchaser was a convicted felon. But only four out of every five firearms purchases occur through the formal process involving a federal firearms licensed dealer.

About 22% of purchases fall into the loophole in background checks that allows individuals to sell person-to-person. This creates the opportunity for many weapons to get into the hands of people who pose a danger. In 2019, state and federal background checks processed approximately 12 million gun sales. Another 3.3 million were likely sold by private sellers without any background checks. By my estimates, assuming the 0.5% rejection rate historically experienced by the NICS system, 17,000 firearms fell into the hands of felons, abusers, or others who would otherwise be prohibited by the Brady Act. And that was just in 2019.

The undocumented teenager who shot Sakran in the neck in 1994 would have failed the background check process had the Brady Act been in place at the time. Only fifteen states and the District of Columbia require background checks on private sales of firearms from one owner to another, according to the Giffords Law Center to Prevent Gun Violence.[6] Virginia, where Sakran grew up and was shot, was not one of these jurisdictions until it closed the loophole for background checks on the private sale of firearms in 2020.[7]

The number of "bad guys with guns" who own firearms without the vetting of a background check may be even higher than my back-of-the-envelope calculation if we assume that current and future criminals selectively choose to obtain their firearms using the loophole of private sales in states without universal background checks. They might also use illicit means such as straw purchases—by which someone who can pass a background check buys a gun and gives it to someone who otherwise would have failed it. Background checks are run only half the time when firearms are transferred through private sales, according to recent evidence.[8] Such imprecise estimates of the numbers of deadly weapons floating around in the hands of people who should not have access to them is a problem.

"We know a lot about the first sale of that gun, and we know a lot about the last person caught with that gun. We just don't know a lot about what's in between," says Harold Pollack, co-director of the University of Chicago Crime Lab.[9] At some basic level, every crime gun starts out as a legal gun. Universal background checks might stall that transition.

Background checks are useful for preventing the loss of life from gun violence. In the 2020 edition of the RAND Corporation's book *The Science of Gun Policy*, moderate evidence shows that background checks performed by federal firearms licensed dealers decrease firearm homicides. However, the evidence for the effect of private-seller background checks on firearm homicides remains inconclusive.[10]

Just because we know that background checks reduce firearm homicides when they are conducted by federal firearms licensed dealers, that does not mean that all private sales should be banned. Otherwise, how could individuals sell guns they no longer wanted? It does suggest that if background checks are to be processed on all gun sales in this country, a federal firearms licensed dealer should be involved.

A 2019 law would have closed this loophole. H.R. 8, the Bipartisan Background Checks Act of 2019, which passed the House of Representatives on February 27, 2019, by a vote of 240 to 190, died on Republican Senate Majority Leader Mitch McConnell's desk while waiting for a vote at the conclusion of the 116th Congress.

Background checks function in tandem with waiting periods. Waiting periods imposed by the Brady Act lasted for only a few years, until 1998, when the NICS came online. Now the FBI completes over 25 million checks annually, with 90% occurring instantly; it only takes 107 seconds to process the average background check.[11]

Two minutes is not enough of a waiting period.

For the 10 percent of cases in which the background check doesn't happen immediately, a three-day waiting period is the default, during which the FBI has time to complete an evaluation of the potential buyer. But after that three-day period, the federal firearms licensed dealer has the option to give the gun to the buyer if the FBI hasn't finished their work.

In 2018, there were over 4,240 transactions in which firearms were transferred from the federal firearms licensed dealer to the purchaser after the expiration of the built-in three-day waiting period imposed by the FBI. Of these transactions, 3,960 guns were placed into the hands of prohibited persons.[12]

It is then up to the Bureau of Alcohol, Tobacco, Firearms and Explosives to retrieve those guns. But how easy would that be, especially if the buyers were intent on harming someone in a rapid time frame? Tragedies like the mass shooting at a Black church in Charleston, South Carolina, illustrate the dangers of what can happen when someone can obtain a firearm after a three-day wait but before a full vetting can be completed.[13] People seeking protection from an abusive partner can be killed prior to obtaining a gun for their own self-defense.[14]

It makes sense to me that we keep the focus on primary prevention—interventions such as universal background checks and brief waiting periods—to stop deadly violence from occurring in the first place. That's the view from public health professionals who advocate for a prudent course of action using what public health experts call the precautionary principle. The evidence supports this strategy. Studies on violent crime reveal that waiting periods may decrease total homicides and firearm homicides.[15]

However, background checks and the brief waits that come with them require that all the necessary data are present to adequately vet gun buyers. In 2017, a 26-year-old man who had been court-martialed by the air force in 2012 shot up a church in Sutherland Springs, Texas. Twenty-six people, including an unborn child, were murdered.

The air force had never reported the information about the court-martial to the FBI. The year after the Sutherland Springs church shooting, Texas Republican senator John Cornyn helped pass the Fix NICS Act, which has resulted in 6 million additional records entering the database.[16] It's designed to prevent further tragedies by ensuring that the background check system has robust and complete data. That means that the military and the criminal justice and health care systems should freely contribute to the FBI database by tearing down silos between these portions of our society and the information flowing into the NICS. Sakran and I, along with fellow gun violence prevention advocate Kyle Fisher, argued for these changes in *Health Affairs*.

Clinicians will not remain silent about firearm-related injuries and deaths, and we will continue working diligently with other stakeholders to provide data-driven solutions to tackle this public health crisis.

If we look back to November 7, 2018, when the NRA tweeted its admonishment of doctors, recall that the NRA argued that if we are to look at research, we should consider the best data available. As practitioners of evidence-based medicine, we know that clinical practice should be determined based on either strong, convincing trials or a constellation of data that point toward similar conclusions. As advocates for evidence-based health policy, we similarly believe that legislation proven to reduce injury and death should be passed and implemented. The NRA suggested that doctors consult the RAND Corporation's Gun Policy Analysis.

We have studied the RAND analysis. The report summarizes the best available research on gun policy. Using a robust methodology, the analysis examined policies and stratified each policy based on a range of evidence strength from "no studies" and "inconclusive" to "limited," "moderate," and "supportive." In the end, the RAND analysis reached several conclusions based on policies reaching the threshold of "limited," "moderate," or "supportive" evidence. Here's what we know works to save lives.

Universal Background Checks.

The data support expanding background checks on all firearm purchases, including private-party transactions, to reduce the likelihood of firearm deaths from both homicide and suicide. This policy has recently received support from the medical community including statements from the American College of Physicians and the American College of Surgeons.[17] The Bipartisan Background Checks Act of 2019 (H.R. 8), introduced by US Representatives Mike Thompson (D-CA) and Peter King (R-NY) has 231 co-sponsors. Currently, 29 states do not require background checks for private handgun sales, and 37 states do not require background checks for private sales on long guns. Allowing universal background checks for nearly all purchases of firearms is an important first step to reducing firearm injury and death in the United States, and 97% of Americans support this policy.[18]

Some of the existing provisions of the Brady Handgun Violence Prevention Act cannot be faithfully executed without the cooperation of the states and local law enforcement. Although studies of states that added mental health checks to the standard criminal background check procedure prior to gun purchases showed a stark reduction in firearm suicides, not all states require complete and timely reporting. Thus, overall enforcement of the mental health background check provisions in the Brady Act is lax. The 10th Amendment prevents the federal government from compelling states to comply with all portions of the Brady Act. Therefore, it is necessary that Congress properly incentivize compliance.

For instance, facilities accepting Medicare or Medicaid payments could be asked to inform the National Instant Criminal Background Check System (NICS) when prohibited persons—those involuntarily committed for mental health emergencies—are admitted. Alternatively, federal grants to states and law enforcement could become contingent upon compliance with the NICS.

In an effort to help enhance the effectiveness of the federal background check system, bipartisan legislation, the Fix NICS Act of 2017, was signed into law by President Donald Trump in March 2018. This legislation requires federal authorities to comply with existing law and report criminal history records to the NICS. It also offers incentives to states that upload felony and domestic violence records in the background check system. . . .

The eyes of physicians, nurses, and health care professionals across the United States have opened to the public health crisis of firearm-related injury and death sweeping across this country. The question is, what will we do now that we are awakened to this issue?[19]

- Background checks performed by federal firearms licensed dealers decrease firearm homicides.
- Waiting periods might decrease total homicides and firearm homicides.

CHAPTER ELEVEN

The Mental Health Paradox

Approximately two-thirds of all gun deaths are due to suicides. Dr. Emmy Betz, an emergency physician living near Denver, Colorado, has had her eyes open to this link between violence and self-harm for some time. She sees at least one or two patients every day who are suicidal. But she realizes the limitations of a medical industrial complex designed to "move the meat," a curt phrase in the satirical novel *The House of God* that described the daily struggle of physicians working inside America's hospitals in the 1970s. The concept of seeing as many patients as possible and moving quickly from case to case is arguably much worse now, half a century later.

Physicians do their best to put patients over profits. But when the metrics look at indices as blunt as "patients seen per hour," it is no surprise that, as Betz says, "I think we do a pretty lousy job of taking care of people with mental health issues in the ER."

Betz, a red-haired emergency doctor in her late forties, says "The system is pretty broken. We don't really know how or what we can do to help them so they just sort of sit there for hours." Amid the coronavirus pandemic, the situation only worsened with patients lingering in emergency departments for days or even weeks. In extreme cases, according to Dr. Chris Kang, a former president of the American College of Emergency Physicians, some individuals with mental health issues have been stuck in emergency departments for over six months.[1]

These patients, who may be suffering from a psychotic crisis due to schizophrenia or a bout of suicidality because of major depression or bipolar disorder, are considered lucky if they receive a moment more than the twelve minutes, on average, a patient gets with an emergency physician.[2] Patients with serious psychiatric concerns sometimes languish for hours or even days as they wait for specialized psychiatric care. This creates a sense of powerlessness among health care workers who become disillusioned with the health "care" system. This leads to burnout, depression, and, in the case of some 400 or more health care workers a year, the end of life by suicide.

Betz copes by spending time outdoors at her family's vacation home west of Denver. She sits outside in the crisp air of the Rocky Mountains, sometimes sipping red wine, sometimes white wine, allowing the majestic beauty of the craggy peaks to dance in front of her eyes. One night, as the sun set over the snowcapped peaks and the amber hues disappeared on the tree-lined valleys, Betz chose to sip on a Manhattan to help detach from her work.

Unplugged from the rest of the world, Betz allowed her mind to drift. It wandered to two personal events that resonate with her current work as a suicide prevention advocate. Decades ago, an uncle she never had the chance to meet died by firearm suicide. His death impacted her family in ways that reverberate to this day. But more recently, in 2017, one of her cousins followed the same path. Betz gathered her thoughts on what she described as one of the worst moments of her life.

Her mother had called. She had news.

For her family's sake, Betz didn't want to tell me her cousin's name when I interviewed her. Momentarily putting herself into his shoes, Betz embraced the emotions he must have experienced. It saddened her when she empathized with how he must have been feeling, trying to contemplate the level of despair, grief, and hopelessness running through his mind.

"Why didn't I do more?" she said, internalizing the anguish, a pain compounded even more by the fact that she is a research expert in the field of suicide prevention. Knowing that her cousin had had mental health concerns for years, Betz felt angry that he even had possession of a gun. As mentioned in chapter 4, nearly 90% of people who attempt suicide with a firearm will die, a risk far greater than with attempts by other means.[3] Betz suspects that her cousin would still be alive and with his family today if he hadn't had access to a gun.

Policy Prescription: Mental Health Checks Do Not Necessarily Save Lives, but Permits and Licenses to Purchase Firearms Do

The National Alliance on Mental Illness reports that one in five adults experience mental illness every year while one in twenty-five people experience a severe mental illness that impairs or limits major life activities.[4]

The Brady Act placed restrictions on individuals with mental illness or intellectual disabilities that are so severe that they have been committed to a mental institution. This is but a fraction of the population of Americans with diagnosed mental illness. However, physicians must always balance public safety—and the safety of our patients—with protection of their human rights and must avoid stigmatizing people who are afflicted with diseases that have resulted in terrible acts against humanity.

Dr. Amy Barnhorst, a psychiatrist at the University of California, Davis, explained the dilemma of trying to judge whether it is reasonable to take away a person's civil rights. "That's the question that psychiatrists, especially inpatient psychiatrists like me, deal with all the time. That's what involuntary commitment is all about. Right? Are you willing to take away this person's civil rights?" she asked rhetorically. "Their ability to, like, roam free in their neighborhoods, smoke when they want to, eat what they want to, wear their own clothes, visit with their friends and family. Are you willing to take all those things away in the name of protecting them from themselves or protecting society from them? Those freedoms to me are huge."

Reflecting on a specific patient of hers who had been involuntarily committed for many years due to his proclivity for violence and the danger he posed to society, she recognized that these restrictions on individual freedoms are the "price you pay for that kind of safety."

For most people, however, involuntary commitment for years is not the norm. Barnhorst remarked that even for people with a diagnosed mental illness, "people slide in and out of good times and bad times all the time." During those times of crisis, it is completely appropriate, from a medical perspective, that firearms could be temporarily removed from people. The difficulty of creating a dichotomy between those who can have guns and those who cannot ignores the dynamism of mental health.

Most states require that either mental health records or court records be submitted to either a state or federal repository so that individuals who would be disqualified due to severe mental health issues would be listed in the NICS database. However, the federal government cannot universally mandate reporting. Following certain tragic incidents, such as the Virginia Tech shooting of 2007, some states have ramped up their own reporting requirements. And as reporting has increased in recent years, the percentage of potential firearms sales that have been rejected due to this particular provision of the Brady Act has risen. Thus, it is reasonable to expect that important outcomes such as firearm suicides would have declined. Unfortunately, the most up-to-date data fail to support that hypothesis.

Researchers who explore the subject of violent crime among individuals with mental conditions commonly note that individuals with mental health issues are much more likely to be *victims* of violent crime rather than perpetrators. Although *The Science of Gun Policy* finds that mental health checks have the beneficial effect of reducing arrests for violent crime, mental health checks do not have a significant impact on either firearm homicides or firearm suicides.[5]

Betz would be mistaken to assume that running a mental health check on her cousin prior to his purchasing a firearm would have saved his life. She remembered that her cousin enjoyed going to the range to shoot. "I feel like it was terrible for him to have one in the home," she said when thinking of her cousin as a gun owner. She was angry that while she was working with gun ranges and firearms retailers as partners and friends in her personal quest to reduce the risk of firearm suicides, "they were why he had had access."

"It's not anything that I've . . . kept a secret," she said. "That was in the midst while I was doing all this work and [I] briefly thought about stopping. . . . Continuing to do this work is probably the best way to honor him."

Betz is attempting to fill the large gap in the National Rifle Association's practices. While the NRA promotes the accumulation of guns in the hands of Americans and offers a firearm safety course, it does not mention suicide prevention. Perhaps it is the "master of my own domain" bravado, a culture and mindset pervasive in the gun community, that causes people to think that a person can control their own destiny by wielding an SIG Sauer, an AR-15, or a Winchester rifle. Such attitudes, however, leave a tremendous gap in discussions of firearm safety when the NRA and other Second Amendment zealots will not even mention, let alone address and confront suicide prevention.

***

In the spring of 2019, I drove from Houston to the Texas state capitol building in Austin to testify on behalf of the Texas College of Emergency Physicians and the Texas Medical Association about firearm safety. There was a bill pending in the Texas legislature, proposed by state senator Carol Alvarado, that asked the state to hold a public awareness campaign on firearm safety and suicide prevention.

This was my testimony:

I have seen countless individuals who have attempted suicide by hanging, stabbing, or taking pills, but only rarely have I seen anyone who made it to the ER after shooting themselves—not because it is uncommon—but because firearm suicide attempts are extremely likely to be lethal. I can recall the case of a young man who pointed a gun at his head, pulled the trigger, and literally blew his brains out the other side of his head.

Unfortunately, this is not uncommon. The United States has the highest firearm homicide and firearm-related suicide rates of all high-income countries.[6] Firearm suicides outnumber homicides nearly two to one.

Texas had more firearm-related deaths—3,353—than any other state, a rate of 12.1 per 100,000 (2016).[7] Physicians are alarmed that suicide is now one of the top 10 leading causes of death in the United States and one of only four causes with significant rate increases. Half of the nation's 44,000 suicides in 2016, more than 22,000, were by firearm. The U.S. firearm suicide rate for people more than 10 years old increased 21 percent from 2006 to 2016 . Like the rest of the country, Texas' suicide rate has increased; our suicide-by-firearm rate of 7.3 is higher than the U.S. rate of 6.5 (per 100,000).

Firearm mortality is the second most common cause of preventable death among U.S. children.[8] The American Academy of Pediatrics reports that most parents believe their children will not touch a firearm or do not know where firearms are kept or can be accessed in the home. But in 2015, 609 Texas children were injured or died by a firearm.

Texas' requirements for the safe storage and security of a firearm are critical to support the prevention of theft or the misuse of firearms by adults and children. We know most parents with firearms in the home will talk to their children about firearm safety, but not all do this—increasing risk in the home. The public health data tell us that children who are with an untrained or otherwise careless adult or a friend with access to a firearm are most likely to be injured or killed in an unintentional discharge.

Keeping firearms away from people who present a risk of harm or who are unable to make sound decisions provides a strong base for managing firearm safety. But having strong state laws on firearm safety will not adequately ensure protection as long as the public is not aware of these requirements or of other measures to reduce firearm accidents and access to firearms for those at risk of harm to themselves. We believe Senator Alvarado's proposal to conduct a statewide campaign on firearm safety and suicide prevention can be an effective measure so the public knows how they can help prevent these injuries and deaths.

We recognize that about 40 percent of the U.S. adults own one or more firearms or live in a home where a firearm is present. My household is one of these. The members of the Texas College of

Emergency Physicians and the Texas Medical Association remain focused on proven prevention and harm reduction methods in all areas of public and population health. Physicians have a role in addressing the public health crisis of gun violence and firearm safety. We will continue to talk to our patients about safety measures in the home. We encourage you to take action to approve Senate Bill 1573, and we offer our assistance with implementation of this important legislation.

Unfortunately, no one heard that testimony. The hearing for SB1573, which I was prepared to testify in favor of on behalf of two medical organizations representing over 55,000 physicians, was cancelled at the last minute because a group of armed Second Amendment fanatics had protested in front of the homes of lawmakers. Where are we as a country when we cannot even allow elected representatives to listen to the research about how to prevent suicides?

"We all have lost people," Betz notes. Some have lost spouses, children, or other loved ones. As physicians we have all lost patients, like an army veteran I treated who blew a hole in his head due to his own self-directed violence.[9] Some of us have lost colleagues.

"I'm not the only one who has those stories," Dr. Betz humbly reflected. "There's still a lot of stigma around talking about suicide." Yet she actively confronts the stigma, actively challenges the problem, and will speak up for the over 23,000 Americans who die by firearm suicide every year. Dr. Betz never stops talking about suicide.

"I'm really grateful to be doing some work with the [Veterans Affairs] and the [Department of Defense] now and looking at servicemembers and veterans and how, you know, particularly in those populations we can help with suicide prevention,"

Betz says. "But I think what I've really been learning from that work is what I alluded to . . . the potential for partnership and collaboration, finding those common solutions that nobody wants to lose loved ones, being able to really work messaging, and understanding how we create effective messages together to move away from gun control and move towards home safety or home security or whatever word we use to describe it."

When opponents of evidence-based solutions to suicide prevention argue against those demanding more gun control, they exploit the fact that the majority of gun deaths are suicides. Perhaps advocates for the Second Amendment think that by neglecting to consider suicides, as stigma about mental illness encourages our society to do, the remaining deaths—largely urban, Black, and Hispanic—become negligible.[10]

It is easier for some people to ignore Black and Brown adolescents, men, and women murdered in Washington, DC; New Orleans; and St. Louis when their deaths are uncoupled from suicides of older, white men in Colorado. In Metro Denver, the levels of urban gun violence are nowhere near what they are in cities like Chicago, Baltimore, or Houston. Firearm deaths in Betz's state of Colorado are overwhelmingly suicides at an alarming rate of three to one.[11] Colorado is far above average in this respect but serves as a great training ground for an injury prevention researcher such as Betz who can focus her energy on a topic that roosts extremely close to home.

Lamenting that people are dying because as a nation we cannot simply be grownups and have a full conversation about violence and suicide, Betz wonders why we continually get sidetracked over how people kill themselves and others. Years ago, she took the National Rifle Association's basic pistol course, firing .22s and AR-15s on the range, but realized that the gun advocacy organization had missed a valuable opportunity to make firearms safer. She founded the Colorado Firearm Safety Coalition because the NRA did not include any suicide prevention opportunities in their discussion of safe use. In the intervening years, Betz has published over four dozen studies on the topics of suicide and guns and is considered by many to be one of the nation's top suicide prevention experts. She believes that the United States needs to culturally adopt the designated driver concept for firearm suicides. She calls her idea "the gun buddy."

What should you do if your gun buddy is displaying signs of depression, hostility, or psychosis? First, gun buddies need to be trained to recognize situations when someone is becoming a threat to themselves. Then they need to be empowered to help their friends. Reducing access to lethal means at a time of crisis can certainly save lives. There is a link between recent handgun purchase and the rate of suicide by means of firearms among purchasers. The risk is 57 times as high as the rate in the general population.[12]

Unlike suicide attempts by strangulation, pills, or cutting, most people will never get a second chance to call 911 when they put a gun to their head. Betz's cousin didn't. Transferring a gun from a person who feels suicidal to a gun buddy could be lifesaving, but in some jurisdictions, it could also be a felony offense. Well-intentioned but poorly written laws inhibit the ability of law-abiding gun buddies to do what is right by their friends and family and temporarily remove a firearm from someone who is at risk of harming themselves. Would you knowingly break that law if it meant saving your friend's life or that of a family member? I would.

Would you do what's right and risk becoming a felon? Or can we go back to our lawmakers and instruct them to rewrite the laws so we can save people's lives? H.R. 8, the gun control law that passed through the Democrat-controlled House of

Representatives in 2019 but stalled in the Republican-controlled Senate in 2020, would have fixed this problem.

Betz doesn't like to deal with the politics of gun policy. She prefers to actively engage her community—gun owners, shopkeepers, and others who have a vested interest in keeping their friends safe from harm. "I wish we could look at this the way we look at car crashes and other things without the political noise," she tells me.

One thing all people need to do if we are to save our friends is to get over the misconception that if we inquire about their mental well-being it will result in their ultimate demise. That is a false way of thinking—a deadly myth. Betz cites research that tells us that simply asking a friend if they are suicidal will not make them kill themselves.

The most important question she asks, one posed to friends, family members, and to her patients, is this one: Do you have access to a gun?[13] It's a question that I, as an emergency physician who routinely encounters patients who feel suicidal, have begun asking. That is why Betz focuses her efforts on gun owners. They constitute a concentrated group of individuals who have the lethal means to harm themselves and can represent one of the easiest groups to intervene with to save lives.

***

Most suicides are impulsive. Nearly half of people who attempt suicide do so within ten minutes of the thought reaching the forefront of their mind.[14]

"Being suicidal is not a terminal illness," Betz notes. Fewer than 5% of suicide attempts result in death.[15] Even among those who attempt suicide repeatedly, only 10% will eventually die.[16] However, among attempts, those conducted by firearms are more likely to be successful. Guns are by far the most lethal means of suicide.[17] In these key studies noted above, the case fatality rate, the rate that people who shoot themselves die from their gunshot wound, was over 80–90%.

Limiting access to means of self-harm can save lives. This concept holds true whether the potential method for a suicide attempt is a chemical pesticide, as was common in Sri Lanka;[18] or carbon monoxide or paracetamol, as in the United Kingdom;[19] or a firearm, as is extremely common in the United States.[20] That's why the analysis from the RAND Corporation's *The Science of Gun Policy* provides some evidence that licensing and permitting requirements prior to purchasing a gun would decrease total suicides and firearm suicides among adults.[21]

Reducing access to the most common and dangerous means of self-harm can save the life of a suicidal person. In order to reduce firearm suicides in the United States, aside from preventing a purchase whenever someone is in crisis, we should have ways to have that individual voluntarily surrender their firearms to a trusted friend, to the police, or to a gun shop owner until the mental health emergency has ended. We could even consider other private sector solutions, such as an Amazon locker or a safe-deposit box where firearms can be temporarily locked away from users who are suffering a crisis.

Betz's solution is simple. "It's just like if a friend has had too much to drink, we hold on to his car keys until he's sober and safe to drive again. In the same way, if someone is troubled and considering suicide, we can work with him to store his gun with a friend or a family member or somehow lock up the gun in the home in a way that he doesn't have access to it."

Involving gun shop owners, especially in smaller towns where a personal relationship between the shop owner and the individual gun owner exists, can serve as a powerful gun buddy alliance. It additionally avoids the complicated nature of using law enforcement as a means of removing firearms from people who are a danger to themselves. Many Americans, especially law-abiding gun owners like lifetime NRA member Dr. Paul Torre, an emergency physician who works with me in Houston's Level 1 trauma center, have a healthy distrust of the government. His interpretation of the Second Amendment is similar to Edwin Leap's; it is the physical means of securing the right to our other, less tangible, liberties.

But Torre, a tall silver-haired man with a strong New Jersey accent, would not want law enforcement or other agents of the state to serve as the means to take a firearm away from a person in a mental health crisis. Using private actors like gun shop owners, as Emmy Betz recommends, provides a reasonable and practical alternative for someone like him. While we wait for the data to accrue from the work that Betz and her team are collecting on the gun buddy concept, we are left to cope with several gun laws enacted in a patchwork of states that demonstrate the ability to save lives by reducing suicide. Although mental health checks are not among these policies, laws that require licenses and permits, institute brief waiting periods, and prevent young adults under 21, adolescents, and children from purchasing or possessing firearms do save lives.[22]

- Mental health checks reduce arrests for violent crime.
- Licensing and permitting requirements prior to a gun purchase decrease total suicides and firearm suicides among adults.

CHAPTER TWELVE

Think of the Children

D r. Eric Fleegler thinks about the thousands of children who would be alive if only America's gun laws were different. Fleegler, a pediatric emergency physician and researcher at Harvard, estimates that "had all of the states had some types of negligence law we would have expected thousands of children not to have died" over a 26-year span.[1] His specific estimate, approximately 4,000 lives saved, means nearly one out of every three firearm deaths in kids up to age 14 could have been averted if laws across the country had been more uniform.[2]

That's where you come in.

All politics is local has been a common refrain for decades now. During the COVID-19 pandemic I saw that *all health care is local*, too. Homicide might be a bigger problem than suicide in some communities; four states—Illinois, Maryland, Louisiana, and Mississippi—have homicide rates greater than suicide rates, according to recent CDC data.[3] But most other communities, like Colorado, where Dr. Emmy Betz practices medicine, face a disproportionate burden of firearm *suicides*.[4] Researchers like her and Fleegler are required to provide the science behind gun violence, but advocates are needed to push for the necessary changes to fix the problem. So what policy tools do we know work to prevent people, especially young people, from losing their lives to guns?

Policy Prescription: The Minimum Age to Purchase Firearms Should Be Raised to 21

George Bernard Shaw famously quipped that youth is wasted on the young. When it comes to gun violence, that adage certainly appears truthful. Just the other day, I held a young man's jaw, the bone crumbling under my grip and blood sputtering from a bullet hole just above his right eye, as I placed a breathing tube into his windpipe to stabilize his airway before the trauma team could take him to the CT scan to assess the extent of his injuries. I have seen countless young men and women like this shot and killed, and each time they appear younger and younger to me.

It amazes me that society will restrict some things, such as automobile rentals, to people by charging a differential rate for those under the age of 25 while we will allow almost anyone to purchase a similarly deadly piece of equipment—a firearm— as soon as they hit the age of 18. In the time that I have been writing this book, firearm deaths have eclipsed deaths from car crashes as the leading cause of death for children and adolescents.[5]

Perhaps there is something that the rental car companies realize about the developing young brain that the framers of the Constitution didn't have the medical knowledge and foresight to recognize. Neuroscientists and car rental companies, however, understand that the development of the adolescent brain into its full, responsible adult form continues until nearly 25 years of age.[6] Thus, many have proposed that all firearms should be restricted to increasingly older and older cohorts. Presently under federal law, handguns cannot be sold by federal firearms licensed dealers to people under 21 years old. However, long guns (rifles) can be purchased once a person reaches the age of 18. In many places, this includes the types of guns implicated in many of our nation's deadliest mass shootings. With the addition New York in 2022 and Colorado in 2023, ten states now require that purchases of any type of firearm be at least 21 years old (see fig. 12.1).

Many people have suggested restricting all firearms sales, especially of semiautomatic center-fire rifles, to people above the age of 21. Firearm aficionado and emergency physician

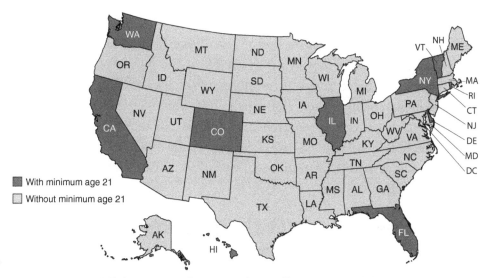

FIGURE 12.1 Minimum Age of 21 to Purchase All Firearms. California, Colorado, Delaware, Florida, Hawaii, Illinois, New York, Rhode Island, Vermont, and Washington require a minimum age of 21 to purchase *all* guns. Washington, DC, and the other 40 states require a minimum age of 18 for gun purchases other than handguns.

Source: https://giffords.org/lawcenter/gun-laws/policy-areas/who-can-have-a-gun/minimum-age/. (January 2024)

Edwin Leap believes that raising the age for anyone who wants to purchase an assault weapon to age 21 is a reasonable and wise policy. The Raise the Age Act introduced by Representative Anthony Brown of Maryland would do that.[7] Detractors might point out that 18 is considered the age of majority for almost everything else in this country, from military service to emancipation from parents. Public health professionals might counter with the understanding that restrictions exist on alcohol and tobacco products to people under 21, even though Americans similarly have a constitutional right to beer, wine, and whiskey thanks to the Twenty-First Amendment! It should be noted that the Raise the Age Act would exclude adults under age 21 who are active military or who are working in law enforcement.

The data from *The Science of Gun Policy* disappoint, though. Although minimum age restrictions on the purchase of firearms by people under 21 can decrease firearm suicides among younger people, such age restrictions won't necessarily stop firearm homicides, unintentional injuries, or mass shootings. Shouldn't we care enough about our youth to do whatever we can to assure that they can live longer, fuller lives without dying by suicide?

Policy Prescription: Child Access Prevention Laws Prevent Deaths

Laws about the safe storage of firearms and ammunition are largely enforced at the state level. Because of this, a patchwork of rules exists across the country. Some states have no laws to prevent child access to firearms, while other states have laws that make it illegal to directly provide a firearm to a child. In some states, the law says that storing a firearm in a manner where a child can use, handle, or, in the most stringent of cases, simply has the opportunity to hold a firearm constitutes negligence.

As many experts and advocates will tell you, the optimal way to safely store firearms would be locked and unloaded so that anyone accidentally coming across them would have to first remove the lock and then load the weapon before it could be rendered capable of causing harm. However, when firearms are purchased for home protection, many Americans choose to leave them out in the open and ready to fire in case of emergency.

When my wife and I first bought our guns, with absolutely no clue how to use them, we did the responsible thing. We went to the range for lessons. Following those lessons and for months afterward, I mentally rehearsed the steps I needed to take in order to convert an unloaded weapon into a killing machine should the need arise. In five steps, I could spring from whatever I was doing and take someone's life with my .40-caliber Smith and Wesson.

Insert the magazine with my right hand. Pull back on the slide. Use my left thumb to drop and disarm the safety. Aim using my dominant left eye. Pull back firmly but steadily on the trigger with my left hand. I have since rehearsed these simple steps in my mind hundreds of times while lying in the bed getting ready to go to sleep. But simple doesn't make it safe.

Knowing what to do doesn't matter when your pulse is racing, your hands are trembling, and there is pressure to perform—whether you are in the trauma bay or the operating room or when someone has breached your property. That's why in medicine we spend years honing our craft. We must have ample opportunities for simulation. That's why police, soldiers, and responsible gun owners, me included, go to the firing range. These skills require the hands and the eye to work in concert with the mind. Guns and the skills to fire them cannot be taken lightly.

Just like you wouldn't hand a scalpel to a child, you should do everything in your power to keep firearms out of the hands of curious children who do not understand their lethal potential. Arthur Kellermann's 1986 paper clarified that firearms provided more peril than protection when present in the home. The science was clear: "For every case of self-protection homicide involving a firearm kept in the home, there were 1.3 accidental deaths, 4.6 criminal homicides, and 37 suicides involving firearms."[8] Every firearm owner must look at these facts and decide for himself or herself whether the benefits of protection outweigh the risk of unintentional or deliberate deaths.

After my home was broken into, my wife and I kept our handgun and shotgun available unlocked but unloaded for that rare purpose. The ammunition was nearby in case I ever needed to defend my home. Looking back on that, it was suboptimal for someone who prides himself on talking about safe storage. Over the years, I've learned that the safest way to store your gun and your ammunition, if your goal is to prevent children from accessing them and harming themselves or others, is to lock them up in separate areas. But we yearned to balance safety from intruders while keeping ourselves safe from the deadly weapon lurking inside the house.

This compromise worked fine until we had a child. One day I witnessed my son, then a precocious four-year-old, grab his small gray wooden chair, slide it up to the mantle, stand on his tippy toes, and grab a remote control so he could change the TV channel to Peppa Pig. I calmly walked up the stairs of our two-level house, the hardwood flooring creaking with every other step, and grabbed my handgun and the two magazines that went with it, moving them from my top dresser drawer and locking them inside our safe. My gun remains there to this day; the risk of family fire is one that I am no longer willing to take.

Child access prevention laws make it a crime on the part of the irresponsible gun owner to leave a weapon out in such a way that a child could grab it and injure themselves or another person. Some states, such as Minnesota, impose penalties on the adult owners when firearms are stored in a negligent manner in which a child *might* access the firearm, even if the child doesn't actually do so. Others, like Texas, impose penalties if the child takes hold of the firearm whether or not an injury occurs. Other states, such as North Carolina, impose penalties only if the child carries the firearm and either commits a crime or injures someone with it.

This patchwork of laws has provided enough variability to create the natural experiments needed to understand which of the various firearm policies has the best chance of improving firearm safety, limiting injuries, and reducing deaths. Recklessness laws, those that penalize adults for directly supplying children with guns, do not save lives; only the more stringent negligence laws have that potential. Twenty-one states and Washington, DC currently have some form of child access prevention (CAP) laws. The other twenty-nine states do not have CAP laws at all (see fig. 12.2).

I'm shocked when I pore over the statistics. Over 4 million American children live in a home with an unlocked and loaded firearm.[9] Most of these children know where these guns are stored, which means they know how to get their hands on them. Up to 90% of firearms used in youth suicides, unintentional shootings, and school shootings come from the home of their family or the home of relatives and friends.[10] Safer storage might prevent up to 300 injuries and fatalities among youth

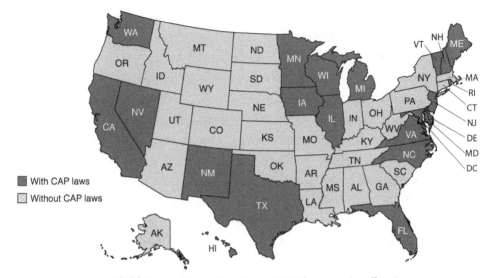

FIGURE 12.2   Child Access Prevention Laws. CAP laws are in effect in Washington, DC, and 21 states: California, Delaware, Florida, Hawaii, Illinois, Iowa, Maine, Maryland, Michigan, Minnesota, Nevada, New Hampshire, New Jersey, New Mexico, North Carolina, Rhode Island, Texas, Vermont, Virginia, Washington, and Wisconsin. CAP laws may differ slightly from safe storage laws which are not addressed here.

Source: https://giffords.org/lawcenter/gun-laws/policy-areas/child-consumer -safety/child-access-prevention-and-safe-storage/. (January 2024)

Note: Child access prevention laws differ slightly from safe storage laws, which are not mentioned in this figure.

each year, based on certain assumptions about the effectiveness of the intervention and the percentage of gun-owning households that switch from keeping loaded, unlocked firearms to locking up all guns.[11]

In his book *Another Day in the Death of America*, Gary Younge describes the harrowing tale of an 11-year-old boy who died from a negligently stored firearm in Michigan, a state that at the time of the boy's death did not have any form of child access prevention law. Tragedies such as that can inspire parents to move their gun from a dresser or a side table or under the bedroom pillow to inside a locked safe and in so doing save their kid's life. But sometimes parents need a nudge. Child access prevention laws can prompt gun owners to take actions that save lives.

I, for one, am tired of turning on the news and seeing the story of a young child shooting and killing a sibling because he or she found a gun that was assumed to be a toy. Nearly half of self-inflicted firearm injuries and unintentional injuries could be prevented if states with weak or without any child access prevention laws adopted strong ones, defined as laws that impose penalties for negligent storage.[12]

Delving into *The Science of Gun Policy* further, the research demonstrates even more beneficial effects of child access prevention laws on a plethora of relevant outcomes important to physicians and parents. There is moderate evidence that child access prevention laws decrease firearm suicide among young people. If we can keep guns out of the hands of young, depressed people who otherwise cannot legally purchase guns themselves, their access to lethal means would decline and so too should their likelihood of completed suicide. Limited evidence suggests that child access prevention laws decrease total suicides among youth aged 14–20 by nearly 10%, and strong evidence indicates that child access prevention laws decrease firearm self-injury among young people. The RAND Corporation analysis also provides some evidence that child access prevention laws reduce firearm assault injuries.[13]

Child access prevention laws demonstrate strong evidence of a reduction in unintentional injuries and deaths among children. Almost anyone would expect that these impacts on children and adolescents would be common sense, but these protective effects might even extend to injuries and deaths in adults. Among the many policy levers available to lawmakers, child access prevention laws are among the best supported by the available evidence to improve the health of the American people. Shockingly, several states still do not have these laws on the books. If you are reading this and you live in one of those states, now is the time to get to work to protect your children or the kids of families around you!

As child access prevention laws still vary widely among states, a remedy has been proposed at the federal level to provide some standardization. Section 305 of the Blair Holt Firearm Owner Licensing and Record of Sale Act, proposed by Representative Bobby Rush of Illinois in 2019, would have provided a federal law making it unlawful for a gun owner to recklessly store a loaded firearm or an unloaded one with accessible ammunition where a child may gain access to it.[14] Enacting this law, known to reduce unintentional injuries, suicides, and firearm assaults, could save the lives of approximately one American boy or girl every day.

- Child access prevention laws decrease firearm suicide among young people.
- Child access prevention laws decrease total suicides among youth aged 14–20 by nearly 10%.
- Child access prevention laws decrease firearm self-injuries among young people.
- Child access prevention laws reduce firearm assault injuries.
- Child access prevention laws reduce unintentional injuries and deaths among children.
- Minimum age restrictions, when implemented for the purchase of firearms by people under 21 decrease firearm suicides among younger people.

CHAPTER THIRTEEN

Under the Gun

The emergency department stretcher rolled into the trauma bay at the University of Chicago, leaving behind a trail of fresh, red blood dripping down the hallway. On it, a 38-year-old Black woman whose beaming wide grin had graced the halls of this emergency department many times before struggled to hold onto life. Dr. John Purakal looked down at his patient, a colleague he had worked with several years earlier when they were trainees. Dr. Tamara O'Neal's empty eyes stared back at him.

Moments earlier, her former fiancé, a man from whom she had sought a protective order, had waited for her in the parking lot of Mercy Hospital, knowing that O'Neal often stayed long after her shift to wrap up care for her patients. As she exited Mercy, a hospital a few miles north of the University of Chicago, he ambushed her in the parking lot.[1] Witnesses inside the hospital heard the first gun shot and watched as the man stood over O'Neal, firing shot after shot after shot after shot after shot into her body as she bled out on the pavement.

After shooting O'Neal, the man ran toward the hospital on a shooting rampage. He struck Dayna Less, a pharmacy resident, and Samuel Jimenez, a police officer, before responding officers landed a bullet in the killer's belly. The killer turned his Glock on himself.

O'Neal, clinging to life, was rushed from the parking lot of Mercy to the University of Chicago Hospital, one of the city's Level I trauma centers. Her friend John Purakal was there to attend to her. "I knew her, trained with her, saved lives with her and tonight, tried to save her life," he said. Despite all efforts, O'Neal died in front of him. "I broke down in front of my coworkers when we lost her. . . . We lost a beautiful, resilient, passionate doc."

As the news broke across the nation, my thoughts immediately turned to several physician friends in Chicago scattered across the various emergency medicine programs in that city, one of whom I knew had previously been in a relationship that had experienced a violent moment.

O'Neal's murder happened a mere twelve days after the National Rifle Association told physicians to stay out of the gun violence debate. Her death solidified my resolve to solve this nationwide problem. The cycle of violence doesn't always end when the shooting stops, and the cycle of violence doesn't always begin when the trigger gets pulled.

The warning signs had been there, an indication that the disease of violence was present but not yet manifest. Perhaps we can also interrupt the cycle of violence in the second phase of prevention—intervening to prevent bodily harm once someone already has a gun.

The nature of intimate partner violence creates a conflict about silence for clinicians. While it is commonplace for us to act as the whistleblower when we suspect abuse of children or of elderly patients who are otherwise unable to care for themselves physically, mentally, or financially, the duty of being a mandated reporter as it exists in those situations does not exist when there is violence between two previously consenting adults involved in an intimate relationship. In some instances, we are even prohibited from warning someone who may be at imminent risk of murder.

In the late 1960s, Tatiana Tarasoff, a student at the University of California, Berkeley, met and briefly dated a man who was a graduate student at Berkeley. Their relationship exemplifies this conflict for physicians. When it ended, the man became depressed. He looked for help from a psychiatrist, describing his intention to hurt and eventually kill the young woman.

When the psychologist attending to the man heard of his plans to harm the young woman, he recommended that the man be placed into commitment, which he was. However, the man was eventually released. He returned to the community, where he befriended and even lived with Tarasoff's brother until he could execute a devious plan during which he stabbed Tatiana Tarasoff to death.

In the aftermath of the killing, which had been foretold to the psychologist, the parents of Tatiana Tarasoff sued the University of California, Berkeley. The case eventually was decided in the Tarasoff family's favor and established something henceforth known as the Tarasoff doctrine: the duty to protect the life of an individual specifically threatened by a patient outweighs the right to privacy expected from the physician-patient relationship. Whenever someone tells me that they want to harm someone else, I feel it is my duty to find out who that person might be.

While the Tarasoff case instantly became the rule in California, the same thing did not necessarily happen in other states. Over time, other states enacted the Tarasoff doctrine as formal statutes that allow doctors to break patient confidentiality rules in order to protect others who might be in danger. In states that accept the Tarasoff doctrine, mental health professionals (or any physician, for that matter) must inform an individual who is at an imminent risk of harm from their patient.[2] Other states, such as Texas, where I practice, do not require that clinicians break the confidentiality of the doctor-patient relationship but permit them to do so when a legitimate threat to another person is present. The federal patient privacy law, HIPAA, allows clinicians to disclose patient information if necessary to prevent imminent harm to the patient or another person.[3] However, a third category of state laws leaves clinicians with moral and legal ambiguity. There is no duty to warn, and there is no protection against violating a patient's privacy if the clinician chooses to warn. It's a "damned if you do, damned if you don't" situation in the worst possible way when an innocent person's life might be on the line.

But what do you do when your patient is already the victim? Should you mandate that she (or he) contact the police? The consensus among those who understand the complexity of intimate partner violence is that the most dangerous time for an abused partner is around the time that he or she plans to leave their abuser. As an emergency physician, I have seen countless people, almost always women, who have been beaten by boyfriends or husbands. Although their physical injuries have been addressed and will heal in time, the most important thing I ask is, "Do you have a safe place to go to?"

Oftentimes it happens to be a relative's house. Sometimes it's a shelter.

In Houston, staff at one of these shelters come and pick up an abused woman from the emergency department, whisking her away to an undisclosed location. It's dangerous even for the physicians and the nurses caring for an abused person to know where their next safe place is because we could personally be threatened by an abuser seeking to do harm to his partner.

Occasionally, a patient who is the victim of domestic violence has nowhere to go that is safe. The only strategy for keeping her safe is admitting her to a bed in the hospital to avoid sending her out into the dark of night or back into a potentially deadly situation. Abused people are forced to return to the situation they are in too many times, a situation made more dangerous by the presence of deadly means such as guns. One of the most difficult parts of our job during these times is avoiding judgment in our voices, our body language, and in our words. If leaving might result in further harm to our patient, who are we to blame her for returning to an abusive situation? Keeping the police out of the situation or returning to an abusive home is sometimes the safest thing for someone involved in the web of intimate partner violence—at least until a more suitable way of escape becomes feasible.

Intimate partner violence, a pattern of behavior between romantic partners or family who live in the same home, can include physical violence, sexual violence, stalking, and psychological aggression. One in four women experience intimate partner violence over the course of their lives.[4] According to one report, 50% of women seen in emergency departments reported a history of intimate partner violence at some point in their lives, of which 11.7% occurred with their current partner.[5] In emergency medicine, we do a poor job of identifying this type of trauma; less than one-quarter of acutely injured victims of abuse are identified as such during their emergency department visit.[6]

The multiple risk factors for death from domestic violence include separating from a romantic partner and a previous history of the partner becoming violent. One of the strongest risk factors is an abuser's access to firearms; it increases the risk of death fivefold.

Domestic violence restraining orders mirror the restrictions on convicted domestic abusers under the Brady background check law and typically require a standard of previous violence. These restraining orders may allow law enforcement to remove firearms from violent people in certain occasions. Such laws have demonstrated that they are effective in reducing the risk of intimate partner homicide. However, the provision that requires the relinquishing of firearms exists in only seventeen states.[7]

Nineteen states and the District of Columbia also have extreme risk protection orders, sometimes known as red flag laws, which, depending on the state, allow family members, health professionals, or law enforcement to petition a judge to remove guns from someone's home if they pose a risk to themselves or others.[8] As these laws are relatively new, there is not great evidence yet as to whether or not they help protect victims of domestic violence.

From 2010 to 2017, the United States witnessed a troubling 26% increase in the number of domestic homicides involving a firearm. America is one of the deadliest places for women around the globe. Women here are more than 21 times more likely to be killed by a firearm than women in other similar nations.[9] And for Black women, like O'Neal, the risk of domestic violence death is, appallingly, twice the rate of such death among white women.

It wasn't inevitable, but the odds were stacked against O'Neal. There were multiple red flags about the danger she was in. Her killer had been kicked out of the Chicago Fire Academy in 2014 for allegedly threatening a female cadet.[10] Earlier that year, his wife had filed for an emergency protective order against him, fearing for her safety. In affidavits, she stated that he slept with a pistol under his pillow and on multiple occasions had pulled it out in a threatening manner, once toward a neighbor, once toward a realtor, and at least once toward her.[11] Despite these terrifying incidents, the protection order limiting O'Neal's future murderer from interacting with his ex-wife lasted for only 16 days. The couple divorced in 2014, citing constant infidelity and abuse as causes, yet O'Neal's killer was not permanently disqualified from obtaining a Firearm Owners Identification Card from the state of Illinois and a concealed carry permit.[12]

Was a firearm necessary for his new career as a security guard in Chicagoland hospitals, where he would eventually meet O'Neal? How could this man, who had a protective order filed against him and whose divorce cited abuse as a reason for ending the marriage, manage to pass a background check that allowed him to legally purchase and carry a 9mm semiautomatic handgun? This man, who had a short temper, poor insight, and terrible conflict resolution skills, was able to stock up on deadly weapons in the years preceding O'Neal's murder.

O'Neal realized these red flags when she decided to leave the relationship. She feared for her safety and called 911 immediately upon seeing her ex-fiancé arrive at her job that Monday afternoon. What would have happened if she had been able to file for an emergency risk protection order prior to that fateful day? Would it have helped? Would she still be alive if he had been forced to surrender his firearms?

The data suggest that such laws implemented in Connecticut have saved the lives of dozens of people whose friends and family thought they were a danger to themselves or others. Those individuals temporarily had their firearms removed and lives were spared.[13]

At the time of O'Neal's death, the Illinois legislature had authorized a similar law that would have permitted law enforcement officers to seize her killer's firearms had she proven that there was a sufficient threat to her safety. However, that law did not go into effect until 42 days after O'Neal breathed her last breath.[14] Perhaps we can save the next person who seeks to escape from a man so filled with rage that he would transmit his anger onto someone else with the deadly flurry of half a dozen bullets.

Policy Prescription: Domestic Violence Restraining Orders Prevent Intimate Partner Homicides When Abusers Surrender Their Guns

Data from the Centers for Disease Control and Prevention indicate that about 20% of all homicide victims are killed by an intimate partner. But of all *female* homicide victims in the United States, 50% are killed by a current or former intimate partner.[15] Toxic masculinity becomes quite apparent when looking at these statistics, and the deadly combination when coupled with guns becomes too much to ignore. Once an intimate relationship becomes abusive, weapons in proximity to the abuser only increase the potential for death.

Research confirms an easily anticipated trend of increased lethality that escalates from the use of fists to the use of firearms.[16] Compared to knives, when guns are were used in a domestic altercation the risk of death increased by over three times; compared to using hands and feet to attack another person, the risk of death with guns was over twenty-three times greater.

Data suggest that whenever a gun is involved in an abusive relationship, the risk of homicide goes up by at least five times for women.[17] For those of us in medicine, especially emergency medicine, Tamara O'Neal's life and death serves as a painful reminder of these statistics.

***

One spring afternoon, as I stood outside our trauma room as the residents tended to a patient, Dr. Brad Scott, the on-call acute care surgeon, and I had a brief conversation on the topic of intimate partner violence. After I mentioned O'Neal, he inquired if I had heard of one of his friends, a transplant surgeon named Dr. Sherilyn Gordon-Burroughs who had worked at Houston Methodist Hospital. She had been shot by her husband.[18] Like O'Neal, Gordon-Burroughs did not live to tell her story. She died in a murder-suicide, leaving behind a young daughter and countless colleagues and trainees grieving from her death.

Of the gun sales denied since the advent of the Brady Act, over 8% were because the purchasers had convictions for domestic violence.[19] However, the criteria that excludes a person from purchasing a new firearm because of domestic violence often requires that they have been married to, have a child with, or cohabitate with the victim. Dating partners, more and more commonly, are the perpetrators of intimate partner violence, yet until the summer of 2022, they were not explicitly subject to the restrictions placed on husbands, wives, co-parents, and cohabitants. This so-called boyfriend loophole was a major flaw in our current firearms policies but was plugged after the school shooting in Uvalde, Texas, when President Joe Biden signed the Bipartisan Safer Communities Act.

The Science of Gun Policy cites evidence that the combination of domestic violence restraining orders, those filed by a victim to keep an abuser away, and regulations that prevent the purchase of firearms and require the relinquishing of currently owned ones can decrease total and firearm-related intimate partner homicides.[20] For people who would be prohibited due to a misdemeanor conviction for domestic violence, laws prohibiting purchase of firearms alone do not appear to substantially impact the risk of firearm homicides. Law enforcement must *remove* guns from the hands of violent people in order for lives to be saved.

What is troubling, however, is that the data reveal a slight relationship between prohibitions associated with stalking misdemeanors and an *increase* in total intimate partner homicides. It suggests that the behavior of stalkers might worsen after they are told to surrender their firearms. For someone like Stephanie Gordy, the trauma surgeon dealing with a stalker, these statistics are frightening. According to one study, living separately from an abuser and owning a gun slightly shields a person from the danger of intimate partner homicide.[21] Instead of trying to disarm her stalker, Gordy has good reason to protect herself with her guns.

- The combination of domestic violence restraining orders, those filed by a victim to keep an abuser away, and regulations that prevent the purchase of firearms and require the relinquishing of currently owned ones can decrease total and firearm-related intimate partner homicides.

CHAPTER FOURTEEN

Violence Interrupted

My phone buzzed in the pocket of my blue jeans one Saturday night at around 10:30 P.M. as the standing-room-only crowd at Minute Maid Park, clothed in vibrant orange tones, erupted in cheers. It was game two of the 2019 American League Division Series playoffs between the Houston Astros and the Tampa Bay Rays. It was taking place a few weeks before I would travel to Denver to meet with Art Kellermann, Megan Ranney, Emmy Betz, Kyle Fischer, and several other firearm injury prevention experts at the annual meeting of the American College of Emergency Physicians. Just as Emmy Betz's personal life and work life had abruptly crossed streams on the day her cousin died by suicide, my work life was soon about to mix with my personal life.

"Lee's been shot," the text from Chelsea Livingston, a medical student at the institution where I practice and teach emergency medicine, read. Lee was my next-door neighbor, an older Black man I chatted with most days when he walked his dogs. I jumped up from my seat and ran to a pair of heavy green metal doors securing a stairwell. I pushed through the doors, entered the stairwell, and dialed the front desk of my ER while a cacophony of hoots at the ballpark got louder.

"Hi, this is Dr. Shinthia," the voice on the other end said. Nashid Shinthia was one of our newer attendings, a short South Asian woman with mocha skin and large round glasses framing her face.

I pressed a finger into my left ear to drown out the noise. "Hey, this is Dr. Dark," I said, relieved that I was talking to someone I had met before. Even though she was new to our department, she was not unfamiliar to me. "One of my neighbors has been shot. Is he over there with you?"

Dr. Shinthia hadn't seen any Code 1 traumas that night, the designation we give to the most seriously injured patients. A Code 1 trauma call activates the entire trauma team, including all the emergency department residents, the emergency department faculty, the surgical resident, and the surgical attending. "But wait, I did hear a page for a Code 1 earlier," Shinthia said. "I think another attending took that one. Let me have them call you back."

I knew I wouldn't hear my phone ring amid the raucous cheers of baseball fans. "Have them text me," I said, walking back to my seat. My wife was high-fiving the fans sitting next to her. I pictured Lee's smiling face. What if Lee is dead? I thought. Who would shoot a nice older guy like him? What had happened on our block while I was at the game?

My wife, a lifelong Houstonian and also an emergency room doctor, had dreamed of moving to Houston's Third Ward ever since she was a girl. The Third Ward with its large and lavish homes, its manicured yards and sculptured hedges, represented the glorious and hard-earned success of Black Houstonians who had not only survived but thrived. Celebrities such as Beyoncé, Super Bowl champion Dexter Manley, and Tony

Award-winning actress Phylicia Rashad have called this neighborhood intersected by the Brays Bayou home. For me, a kid who grew up in the suburbs of Washington, DC, arriving in the Third Ward meant that my family had made it, that years of exams and long hours and debt had finally paid off.

We had arrived in Houston during a typical 100-degree summer in 2013 and moved into a home a few doors down from Lee. The house had been built in the 1940s, a time when Jewish people, excluded from wealthier parts of Houston, had created an enclave that was considered by some to be the Jewish River Oaks. River Oaks remains one of the wealthiest neighborhoods in Houston, featuring luxurious homes, designer shopping, and an air of exclusivity. Third Ward sought to emulate those palatial homes with residences on large lots nestled along the bayou. Following World War II, the Third Ward began to desegregate, but racial tensions flourished. One of the first Blacks to move into the neighborhood, a cattleman named Jack Caesar, had his home bombed with four sticks of dynamite by two white men. In the 1950s and 1960s, the Jewish people in the Third Ward, especially in the homes around MacGregor Way, moved upstream from Brays Bayou, leaving the neighborhood to become what *Texas Monthly* magazine writer Lawrence Wright described in 1982 as "the richest, stateliest, black neighborhood in Texas."[1]

Our two-story house had been freshly renovated; the newest home on the block to receive a makeover as people who had lived here during the preceding decades began to move out of the city or will the property to children who no longer wanted to live so close to downtown. Lee, a man in his mid-50s at the time, was happy to see a young Black couple move into the neighborhood to buffer the waves of gentrification that were on the horizon. Like many of the residents on our street, Lee was an older Black man who had seen the neighborhood change over the course of his years. He had grown up in the Third Ward during the 1960s and 1970s, a time when Black doctors, lawyers, and business tycoons congregated in the large homes along the bayou. He moved to Los Angeles, California, in 1985 to pursue a career in the entertainment industry, doing everything from driving a limousine to operating a news camera, but ultimately returned to the Third Ward to help care for his elderly mother in 2011. Houston's Third Ward was Lee's true home. His block was now my block.

In our morning talks, Lee had told me about the wealthier white families who had been buying property, lauding our neighborhood's culture and history and driving up the cost of living, making it unaffordable for many Black families who had called the Third Ward home for generations. White folks felt that the neighborhood was getting safer, Lee said, but these streets weren't entirely protected from violent crime. One spring afternoon, another neighbor's lawn man was robbed at gunpoint for his leaf blower. I came home from work one night in 2014 to find someone had broken into my house, and in 2015 a man was shot dead in the parking lot of Good Hope Baptist Church, a few minutes' walk from our block.[2]

At the game, the Astros put another run on the scoreboard, causing my wife, a fan of all things Houston, to jump out of her seat in celebration. My mind was racing, distracted by the potential route of a bullet through Lee's body.

If he had been shot distal to the knee or elbow, the speakers in the emergency room would have rung out with a Code 2 announcement, letting staff know that the bullet had missed vital organs and that the senior surgeon, someone like Stephanie Gordy, could stay in the operating room while her surgical residents examined the patient.

But if Lee was struck higher up, proximal to the knee or the elbow, it would have been called out as a Code 1 trauma. Was he hit "in the box," that precious area containing the vital organs of the chest and belly? Almost everyone shot in the box needs some type of surgery to reinflate a collapsed lung, repair critical blood vessels, or explore the bowels in case the bullet has pierced the gut, forcing undigested food and feces into the abdomen.

In my mind's eye, I traced the course of Lee's major blood vessels, the pulsing aorta as it curves from the top of the heart and heads downward toward the major organs—liver, kidneys, and spleen. If these had been hit by the bullet, he could have bled to death at home even before an ambulance arrived, much like my cousin Robbie.

The stadium crowd was erupting into cheers again when my phone buzzed with another text from Chelsea.

Ping! "Heard Lee and his brother got into a fight in Lee's garage and his brother shot Lee in the leg."

Okay, so Lee hadn't been shot in the box, but what if his femoral artery had been ruptured by the bullet? It is still quite possible to bleed to death from a wound rupturing a large blood vessel like that. I immediately thought of Sean Taylor, the Washington NFL player who was shot in the groin by a man during a home invasion. The bullet hit Taylor's femoral artery, the main artery of the leg, and he bled profusely, dying the following day. Was Lee struck like that?

Bullets don't move through the human body smoothly. Whenever a high-velocity projectile enters the skin, it begins to slow dramatically upon impact with bodily tissues, not only distributing its kinetic energy to the tissues it comes into direct contact with but also converting its energy into the form of a shock wave. This shock wave, or cavitation effect, can cause damage to vital structures out of the direct path of the bullet that can be just as bad, if not worse, as the damage to the tissues along the bullet's known trajectory. Not only that, but bullets don't just penetrate the skin and travel in a straight line, like an arrow or a knife; they tumble, they fragment, and they can ricochet, spreading their deadly force in any direction imaginable. In the trauma bay, we often have to go searching with X-rays to identify the resting place of a bullet that began in one place and lodged somewhere unexpected.

Two physical properties determine the amount of energy a bullet can carry to its intended victim—its mass and its velocity. Mass, or how much a bullet weighs, is an easily understood concept in terms of delivering the impact of a bullet. A smaller projectile, like a .22-caliber round, will deliver significantly less punch than a .45-caliber bullet.

Once, a particularly lucky man crossed my path in the trauma bay. He arrived having been shot in the forehead. To everyone's surprise, as the man rolled in on the EMS gurney, he was sitting and laughing with the paramedics. Perhaps he was as hardheaded as he claimed; the .22-caliber round aimed at his skull hadn't been heavy enough to penetrate the bone.

The greater factor influencing the energy a bullet carries to its target is its velocity, or speed. The formula for kinetic energy squares the velocity of the projectile, imparting exponentially greater force to a projectile with a similar weight that is delivered in a faster manner. The bullet that fires from the AR-15, the .223, is similar in diameter and in some instances in weight to a .22-caliber handgun round. However, the velocity of the projectile fired from an AR-15 can be nearly three times as great. The energy imparted into that bullet, therefore, is nine times as great as one fired from a handgun.

While my patient survived the shot to the forehead from a .22 pistol, a single AR-15 round—with an order of magnitude greater energy—could have blown a hole in his skull big enough to reach inside and scoop out the rest of his liquefied brain.

Chelsea couldn't figure out where Lee had been taken. I was stuck playing the part of an anxious friend instead of my preferred role: the doctor equipped with details and answers. I slid my phone into my pocket and rubbed my thighs with my palms; they had begun to sweat from nervousness.

Houston houses the world's biggest medical complex, a miniature medical city within a city that was only a 10-minute drive from the stadium where I was sitting feeling worried instead of entertained. The Texas Medical Center houses 44 institutions and more than 100,000 employees and hosts at least 7 million patients and visitors each year. To which of these places had the ambulance taken Lee? Who was caring for my friend? There were only two viable options—Ben Taub and Memorial Hermann—the city's only Level 1 trauma centers, situated adjacent to one another and just a couple of miles from our houses.

My wife turned and smiled as the Astros scored again, but I couldn't bear to share my anxiety with her as she beamed, not when there were so many unanswered questions. However, she could sense my unease. The smiles on her face wrinkled. I texted Lee's phone, hoping he might respond if he wasn't seriously injured.

He didn't respond.

All night long there was no news. We drove home after a victorious game for the Astros and I parked my car and gazed down the street toward Lee's house, wondering exactly what had taken place there.

Sunday came and went.

I dressed my son, went to church, and still no word from Lee. My neighbor's house sat empty. And then, late on Monday night, I got the news. The bullet had broken Lee's leg. Surgeons had placed a titanium pin inside the shattered bone and Lee was in recovery.

He finally texted back.

Ping! "Thankful to be alive," said Lee. After 48 hours of a tight chest, I could finally exhale. Except it wasn't that simple. Lee had a broken femur that needed fixing in an operation.

Lee's case, as is true for many survivors, provides a living witness to the physical consequences of gun violence—broken bones, chronic pain, paralysis, traumatic brain injuries. For others, the damage hides itself deeper in the form of post-traumatic stress, depression, anxiety, and other mental health issues. And for some, rage and retribution. Recovery can take a lifetime, if it ever arrives. And death, while not immediate, can still result years or decades after a nonfatal firearm injury, as it did for Reagan's press secretary, James Brady.

For James Brady, the bullet that destroyed vitally important parts of the brain that control movement instantly led to paralysis. That paralysis led to other complications such as blood clots forming in the paralyzed limbs that, if they had broken off, could have traveled to the heart and lungs, resulting in serious illness and perhaps death. Others I have seen with traumatic brain injuries or spinal cord injuries from gunshot wounds can develop skin breakdown and urinary retention, each of which could lead to repetitive bacterial infections. Over time, as that person has more and more contact with the health care system, the pathogens swimming in the urine in their bladder change from the normal *E. coli* that characterizes the typical uncomplicated urinary tract infection into one of the more dangerous multidrug-resistant superbugs that breed and thrive in the hospital setting. One day, an infection begins that physicians don't have an available treatment for; this can kill the patient. When this happens, forensic pathologists trace the cause of death all the way back to the bullet that ripped through the patient's brain or spine. It might take decades and a drug-resistant bacterium to do it, but that patient's death gets labeled a homicide. Because without ever being shot, without being paralyzed, without pulmonary embolisms, decubitus ulcers, or urinary tract infections, that person wouldn't have died like that.

***

A few months after the baseball season had ended, I bumped into Lee sitting out on his front porch taking in some fresh spring air. The unseasonably warm Texas sun beamed onto the southern exposure, lighting up Lee's dark brown skin. Mocha, Lee's aging little chocolate-colored Boykin spaniel, greeted me as I approached the house, her wagging tail revealing that the threat of her constant barking was merely a ruse. As I sat with Lee on a bench, we caught up about the World Series. That year, it pitted the Astros against my hometown team, the Washington Nationals.

As a warm winter sun reflected off the muted yellow tones of Lee's house, we reminisced about the playoffs, agreeing that A. J. Hinch, the disgraced Astros manager, had pulled pitcher Zack Greinke out of game seven just a little too early. I was probably the only person in Houston who seemed satisfied with that managerial misstep. Our conversation eventually shifted to the night Lee's brother shot him in the leg. While I looked at Lee's healing brown skin, held together by several black nylon stitches, he described the events of that night.

"I had worked Saturday," Lee recalled while Mocha sat in the grass at our feet. "Five in the morning to 5 o'clock at night at the East Water Purification Plant." After a long day as an operator at a plant where water was purified from muddy sludge, Lee planned on coming home and sitting down to watch the baseball game. He got back to his home just in time to catch Gerrit Cole hurl the first pitch. As one can imagine, work at a plant that processes sludge is dirty work. So after getting home, he tossed his clothes into the washing machine in the garage nestled in the back of the property.

His twin brothers, Rodney and Ronald, who are five years younger than Lee, were also in the home they have shared since their mother died a few years ago. During a break in the action in the second inning, Lee got up to move his car from the narrow single-lane driveway so his brother Rodney could pull his car out. Looking toward the garage, he noticed that all his uniforms were dripping wet, having been pulled out of the washing machine by someone else. He placed his items in the dryer.

Ronald, Lee's other brother, came storming out of the den. Ranting and raving, he burst through the patio and out the gate in a rage. Ronald started exclaiming: "You stealing from me! You're stealing my laundry detergent!" Ronald then made a move to pull Lee's clothes from the dryer.

Lee approached him aggressively, and when Ronald reached down to pick up the laundry, Lee lunged. The two wrestled with each other until Lee had Ronald on his back under the shelves. He started to choke him.

The sun that was rapidly setting behind the houses across the street was sending shadows deep into Lee's driveway, making it more difficult to see. Scuffling in the garage amid dissipating sunlight, Ronald tripped over a pink roll of fiberglass insulation. Stumbling to his feet, he reached into his pocket. He pulled out a gun, quickly aimed it at his brother, and pulled the trigger.

"I knew I was shot, not from feeling it initially, but the way that my leg flew out from under me," Lee told me. "My leg had really, uh, jackknifed under me." He lay on the floor of his garage, starting to bleed from his right leg, with his legs folded like children sit in kindergarten, cross legged. Surprisingly, he didn't feel pain, but anger began to bubble up from inside him.

"Motherfucker, you shot me!" Lee shouted.

"Don't talk to me like I'm a child," the younger brother asserted. "I'm not a child." Then he walked out of the garage and back into the house as darkness covered the scene.

Lee watched his warm, red blood pooling beside his leg and figured it would be best to maintain his position in case moving might further tear or open up a severed blood vessel. In the growing darkness, he could see his neighbor Monique across the street. So he gave a good effort to whistle. But unlike those people whose whistles can attract attention from yards away, Lee's was a soft, feeble noise only audible to himself. Then, nervously, he started to feel the pulsations of his own heartbeat.

"I was excited, but I wasn't going to be excitable," he told me. He started to pray the Lord's Prayer. In his mind he heard the spirit within him calling: Yea, though I walk through the valley of the shadow of death, I will fear no evil: for thou art with me; thy rod and thy staff they comfort me.

"Motherfucker, go get my phone!" he yelled out when he saw his brother pacing nearby. Ronald, the brother who had just shot him, went in the house, crept into Lee's room, and retrieved his phone. Standing over him outside, he threw it down at Lee and wandered off again. He could have ended him right there—another shot to the chest or one to the head—if he had wanted to. Lee lay helpless on the floor of his garage, slowly bleeding from his broken thigh. He dialed 911.

Then he waited.

Soon after, Ronald came back outside from the house carrying two large towels. He threw them down next to Lee and walked away without muttering a word. Sitting there, sopping up his own blood yet unable to move away from it, Lee thought to himself: I don't want to die on the floor in the back of this garage. Within a few minutes, he could see the red and blue lights reflecting off the house across the street. Four police officers exited their black-and-white Houston Police Department cruisers and stationed themselves on the driveway. Lee, unable to move and hidden in darkness, watched as Ronald approached them, setting the scene.

"He assaulted me," Ronald asserted. "Broke my jaw." One of the officers sauntered slowly to the garage, bent over, and looked at Lee. He asked what had happened.

"I'm shot," Lee replied matter-of-factly, twisting his face in disbelief of the police officer's naïveté.

"Who shot you?"

"That knucklehead you were just talking to," he said, pointing a bloodstained finger at his brother.

"He got a gun?" the cop asked. Then, in what seemed like the blink of an eye, the cops tackled Ronald. It was immediate and swift.

The officer tending to Lee took his belt off, wrapping it around Lee's upper thigh as a tourniquet as the paramedics rolled their yellow-and-black stretcher down the driveway to the garage. The paramedic and a cop lifted Lee off the hard ground, settling him onto the transport stretcher. Then they proceeded to cut off his favorite pair of basketball shorts.

"All my privacy is out!" Lee protested. "You can't take me out like this!" By this time, Lee's neighbor Monique had finally barged her way past the police into the area between the house and garage. She had a look of horror on her face. Lee asked her to grab his wallet as they were pushing the stretcher up the driveway. The paramedics shoved Lee into the ambulance, as three neighbors, Sue, Monique, and Saide, pressed up into the entrance. With no shirt on and his shorts immodestly removed, Lee kept both his hands covering himself. Monique tossed the wallet onto the stretcher as they sealed the ambulance doors. The lights began to flash and the siren began to wail, and Lee reflected on his condition. He felt embarrassed and ashamed that he, by getting shot, had brought that kind of attention to the neighborhood.

"We weren't raised around violence," he told me. "To have them out at 9 o'clock at night. To have police in front of my house." That was the shame that ran through his mind. "My mother lived here for 30 years. I've never put myself in harm's way like this," he thought.

The paramedic, a stocky Black guy, jostled him back to reality as the ambulance crossed over Highway 288, the modern dividing line between the Third Ward and the Museum District. He asked, "Do you want to go to Ben Taub or Memorial Hermann?"

Thinking that it was a Saturday night and Ben Taub would be extremely busy, Lee mumbled, "I better go to Memorial Hermann."

"That's a good idea," the paramedic responded.

By the time they finished that brief conversation, the two-mile trek between Lee's house and Memorial Hermann in the Texas Medical Center was over. Sirens off, they unloaded the ambulance and rolled into the trauma bay.

Once inside, the trauma team looked Lee over head to toe, searching for additional wounds during what is called the Golden Hour of Trauma—a time when life-threatening injuries must be found and stabilized. They rolled Lee on his side, looking to see if there was an exit wound on the back of his leg. As they were doing this, he thought, "I could have been shot in the gut or in my privacy or in the chest or in the head." He was blessed that it had only been once in the leg.

Appearing seemingly out of nowhere, Dr. Dave, an orthopedist dressed in all-black scrubs, said: "Man, we are gonna stabilize that leg." By now, Lee's friend Tony had arrived, and as no other life-threatening injuries had been identified, they allowed him to watch as Dr. Dave and his team tended to Lee's shattered femur.

The orthopedic surgeon picked up a power drill that looked to Lee like something just purchased from Home Depot. After anesthetizing the leg with a few shots of lidocaine, Dr. Dave started drilling through the skin, past muscle, through the end of the broken bone, and pushing to the other side. The drill didn't immediately come out through the skin on the other side; instead it tented the skin outward.

Lee watched intently, amazed that he felt no pain, as Dr. Dave tried to get the drill to emerge from the other side of the leg. As Lee glanced over at Tony, he noticed that his friend was starting to take on a slightly different hue.

"I think I saw some steam coming up out of the drill," Tony quipped, although he was green in the face.

Once through to the other side, the orthopedists placed a pin through the far end of the broken bone and began to set some traction on it to stretch out the leg, overcoming the spasm in the thigh muscles.

"You're gonna feel a little tug," one of them said as counterweights were added one by one. After a few had been placed, the counterweights slipped off the bed, tugging fiercely at Lee's leg. That little tug turned into a big yank. It wasn't painful for him, but it did feel like his leg was being pulled apart. In reality, with his bone broken into several pieces, the top and bottom halves of his thigh were being pulled apart. Lee overheard a small laugh from the group of doctors tending to the counterweights at the foot of his bed.

Not too long after having his leg stretched and splinted, Lee was taken to his room on the orthopedics floor, where his roommate, a man from megachurch pastor Joel Osteen's Lakewood Church, had fallen and broken his hip. At close to 8 A.M. on Sunday, they informed Lee that he would be going for surgery around noon. An avid Houston sports fan, Lee thought, "I'm fittin' to miss the Texans game." His roommate was talking incessantly and Lee had not been asleep for hours since the shooting. Time seemed to drag. Eventually, Lee was moved to pre-op, where a team of two nurses wiped his entire body down with what appeared to be medical grade baby wipes.

With his arm pinned behind his head, one of the nurses opened her mouth, gold teeth flashing, and said, "Raise your arms up!" Her voice dissolved into a mix of music playing in the operating room. When Lee opened his eyes up to her again, it was already 3:30 P.M.

The surgery had been successful. "Man, you're gonna do well," Dr. Dave declared before walking out of the room to continue his rounds on his other patients. That quickly, the immediate ordeal was over and the road to recovery had begun.

As an emergency physician, it is not often that I get to hear the full story of someone's misadventure with gun violence. Too often, my patients are dead on arrival, my interaction occurring with a family whose very existence is about to change forever. Or my patients are so sick that they get rushed to the operating room so surgeons can provide damage control to the wounds. While I might follow up on them later, it's not like walking down the street and getting flagged down by your friend who is stuck sitting on his front porch with his walker, unable to explore beyond his front yard.

Lee had not been exposed to violence as a child, despite growing up in an area of the city that is now assumed to have higher-than-average crime rates. Other people are not so lucky. Why are some people pushed toward a lifestyle of violence while others venture out and become successful? In the book *Wrong Place, Wrong Time*, Dr. John Rich tells the story of a young Black man from the Boston area who describes why violence appears as a reasonable option for some men: "If you want to avoid being a sucker, you have to have a rep. If you want to have a rep, you have to earn it. You earn a rep by putting in work. In Jimmy's world, work means doing violence. Having a rep, even if you got it by violence, makes you known. When you are known, you are somebody. . . . Violence worked in his world to accomplish something all of us wanted—to be somebody."[3]

Lee didn't need retaliatory violence to validate his existence. He already was somebody; he had already made a career for himself as a video cameraman for a news channel in Los Angeles. Sitting in his hospital room, Lee remembered that he was angry. But he wasn't lusting for revenge. While for many young men that disease of anger might manifest in continued violence, it was unlikely for Lee. He was older, wiser, calmer. He knew how to cope with his anger.

Too often our society does not work on eliminating the disease agent—hate, anger, and depression. We focus on other strategies to interrupt the chain of infection; that is, the cycle of violence.

Primary prevention for gun violence aims to stop people who shouldn't have firearms from buying or possessing them—felons, fugitives, and abusers. Secondary prevention means removing firearms from an imminently violent person or a suicidal person. It also means protecting portals of entry with bullet-proof backpacks and active shooter drills. When that fails and bullets have pierced the skin, we rely on advances in our trauma care systems to minimize injury once it occurs. This boost to our host defenses represents a type of tertiary prevention; that is, treating the disease of *violence* after it occurs—after the trigger is pulled.

But there is still one last act of tertiary prevention we can provide to people who survive their bullet wounds during what some people call the *second* golden hour of trauma.

CHAPTER FIFTEEN

The Second Golden Hour of Trauma

Some diseases cannot pass from person to person without a vector—whether it be the mosquito or the bullet—to carry it from one person to the next human host. In America, violence, not malaria, is endemic. Guns are a prominent and potent vector for violence, unlike in other parts of the world. Lavaniel "Lee" Henderson never sought to return violence with violence upon his younger brother, Ronald, who had shot him in the leg. People like Lee who have learned to work out differences and find nonviolent ways to resolve conflict are less likely to perpetuate the cycle of violence.

"Conflict's not avoidable, but violent conflict is," said Dr. Rob Gore, a Brooklyn emergency physician, in a 2018 interview with CNN.[1] His refrain is a reminder that violence isn't inevitable. Many cities around the globe can attest to the benefits accrued from programs like his, the Kings Against Violence Initiative, that serve young victims of violence.

In the early 2000s, Glasgow, Scotland, at the time the murder capital of Europe, established a Violence Reduction Unit to stem the flow of blood in and around the city.[2] Homicides totaled 137 in the year 2004, a startling number to experts there for a city of just 600,000 residents, prompting a shift in strategy from policing to public health.

In the decade that followed, homicides reduced by more than half. How did the Violence Reduction Unit accomplish this goal? Gang members, who were responsible for much of the violence, were actively engaged and provided alternatives such as youth clubs, training, and work. Surgeons, who bore witness to the carnage, used their anecdotal experience to inform research. Science ultimately informed policies such as increasing prices on alcoholic beverages to reduce the likelihood of excessive consumption. Alcohol, which had been associated with a large proportion of patients seeking care for assault as well as with the perpetrators of those crimes, became a target for decision-makers working to reduce violence. Authorities used schools to educate young people about bullying and the day-to-day actions they could undertake to prevent escalation to violent confrontation.

None of these actions required regulatory or legislative activities limiting access to firearms. In fact, guns were not even the problem in Scotland. The most common weapons were knives. Like guns, knives were merely a vector in the transmission of the disease. Using a public health approach to address violence, the researchers successfully reduced harm among youth in their community.

These were lessons adopted from colleagues in Boston, Massachusetts, a similarly sized city, which housed a 1990s program known as Operation Ceasefire.[3] Operation Ceasefire began in Boston to address youth homicides, which had been rising in the late 1980s and early 1990s. The city averaged over 40 youth homicides annually prior to the initiation of the program, but after Operation Ceasefire had been in operation for two years, youth homicides decreased to only 10 per year—a 75% reduction in fatalities. However, once the program ended, youth homicides began to rise again, eventually surpassing the previous annual average.

Similar programs that followed the same patterns as Operation Ceasefire—multiagency and interagency collaboration, research, assessment of the nature of violence, continuous adaptation of the program following implementation and impact evaluations—have demonstrated reductions in homicide rates ranging from 34 to 63%. No wonder this simple program from Boston has migrated to Los Angeles, Providence, Chicago, Nashville, Cincinnati, Indianapolis, and across the Atlantic Ocean.

Programs like these, focusing on the intersection of law enforcement with the communities they serve and with the perpetrators of crime, have been adapted to the clinical setting in programs commonly called hospital violence intervention programs. These programs engage clinicians—nurses, social workers, physicians, and surgeons—to translate public health principles to the bedside and thereby find ways to disrupt the cycle of violence and provide lasting benefits directly to their patients and indirectly to the communities they come from.

Hospital violence intervention programs demonstrate the potential to fix the person, the reservoir, in which feelings of hate, retribution, and anger reside. By attending to the reservoir, clinicians can prevent violence from breaking out and spreading to the next person. Gore, who founded a violence intervention program in New York, says that "hurt people hurt people." His program, the Kings Against Violence Initiative (KAVI), stands in the gap to heal hurt people so they do not feel the necessity to hurt anyone else.

Gore, who has a bespectacled brown face and a salt-and-pepper goatee, founded KAVI in 2009.[4] The program grew from a local hospital and community violence intervention program to one adopted by the New York municipal hospital system—the largest public hospital system in the United States.

As academic emergency physicians, Gore and I teach others about the golden hour of trauma: the first hour after an injury is when physicians have the greatest ability to alter the course of our patients' lives. If someone is not killed in the immediate aftermath of a devastating car wreck or from a bullet to the brain, we have a chance to save them in the hospital during this golden hour. The dithering response of the police in Uvalde, Texas, perfectly illustrates how the golden hour is best, or in that case worst, used. Dr. Gilberto "Gil" Arbelaez—the only emergency physician on shift at Uvalde Memorial Hospital the day of the school shooting—never had a chance to save the life of his first patient from Robb Elementary. "She was completely exsanguinated by the time she got to us," he said.[5] The golden hour of trauma is when hemorrhage, or the loss of blood, needs to be stopped and injuries fixed so the road to recovery can begin.

If a patient survives the golden hour, their recovery can become complicated. Infections and organ failure can set in, leading to a person's ultimate demise. However, those events happen outside the immediacy of the trauma bay, outside what Gore and Arbelaez deal with in the emergency department, and outside what we often hear about on television shows.

Gore conceptualizes the *second* golden hour of trauma, a time that, if approached the correct way, can help reduce the likelihood of repeat trauma. Could it be that an early intervention in the hospital might prevent retaliation once a patient returns to their community? Could the provision of psychosocial resources for people who experience interpersonal, daily violence—resources that are typically made available to victims of mass violence like school shootings—provide the substrate needed for the emotional and mental healing of shooting victims while the hospital milieu provides for their physical healing? That is where programs such as KAVI demonstrate their greatest potential for impact.

KAVI exists to disrupt the cycle of violence. Its three planks—school-based, hospital-based, and community-based outreach—aim to find young people where they are in life, whether that means being bullied in school, being assaulted and crossing the path of physicians in the hospital, or recovering in their homes and in the streets. KAVI has reached hundreds of kids, teaching them about conflict resolution and helping them develop coping skills necessary to combat their traumas. These skills facilitate addressing and de-escalating conflict rather than perpetuating it. To build safer, stronger communities, Gore's program helps these young men and women become active young leaders.

Anecdotally, KAVI has demonstrated a reduction in criminal behavior, a much-desired outcome. Published data from other violence intervention programs bear out a fortunate truth; they can prevent trauma recidivism. Aborting this cycle of violence requires hospital-based programs and community-based violence intervention programs that intercede in the situations that inflame the victims and the perpetrators of violence. Recognizing these facts, the Biden administration recently announced investments in community violence-intervention programs such as KAVI.[6]

***

At "The Prince," an affectionate moniker for the Prince George's County Hospital in Cheverly, Maryland, Dr. Kyle Fischer, an emergency physician, witnesses the daily toll of urban gun violence. The Prince serves a predominantly Black community in the suburbs of Washington, DC.[7]

I grew up in Prince George's County and although, as I've told you earlier, it is recognized as having several of the most affluent Black communities in the nation, gun violence is common there, just as it is in my new home of Houston's Third Ward.[8] Decades of gentrification, which pushed people out of Washington, DC, and across the Anacostia River into Prince George's County, brought with it worsening levels of crime and violence.

I sat down with Fischer over a light breakfast of coffee and a blueberry muffin while he recalled a memorable story from his time in residency. Fischer, whose light brown hair sweeps left to right across his forehead, trained in Philadelphia at Drexel University's Hahnemann Hospital, a famed institution that was situated at one of the busiest intersections in all of Philadelphia—the corner of Broad and Vine Streets.

Hahnemann looked a lot like most other typical county hospitals, dressed in unassuming shades of brown and beige. Its emergency department, laid out like a large horseshoe, housed a modern trauma bay that was located right by the ambulance entrance. That was all before a private investor sold the hospital, displacing hundreds of physician trainees, to make way for luxury condominiums.[9]

"When I was a resident in Philly, at Drexel, Hahnemann, I was a senior and I was running around the ER taking care of 10,000 people," he started hyperbolically. "One of the security guards tapped me on my shoulder, and said, 'Hey doc, someone outside said they got shot.' So I quickly ran out to the trauma bay and I saw there was a car with a young kid in the back seat. It was like a little Toyota Corolla. And looked in, it was really dark, so all I could see was a little, you know, enough of a glimmer to know he was shot in the belly. So I ran back in, called level one trauma. They started coming to get him, got a stretcher to get the kid into the trauma bay, but he was too shockingly scared to get out of the car to get taken care of. He was, like, ready to bleed out in the back of the car and was just paralyzed by fear, and we ended up taking him by his arms and legs and throwing him in the stretcher."

Along with the rest of the trauma team, Fischer rushed the young man, who he estimated weighed about 150 pounds, to one of the trauma rooms in the emergency department. Inside his head, Fischer calculated how much medicine would be needed in case the patient collapsed in front of him, needing to be intubated, put on a ventilator, and resuscitated.

"We got in the trauma bay and did all the usual stuff," Fischer continued. They swiftly cut off his jeans and bloody t-shirt, stripping the young man naked so that they could examine every inch of his skin for bullet holes. "I intubated him and he went to the OR."

"I remember the next day I went to look for the news report about what happened with this kid." Back then, in residency, Fischer used to check on all his patients after they presented for a major trauma. "Of course, there was no news report. There's never a news report about our patients," he said despondently.

I can barely stand to watch the news. After I see yet another Black man or woman roll into the trauma bay in Houston, lifeless, blood soiling their clothes and pouring out of the holes in their body, I cannot put myself into the situation of having to relive that trauma after leaving my shift. I quietly whisper inside my head "another life wasted" when someone who looks like me gets brought in dead on arrival as yet another casualty of this uniquely American epidemic. The last time I looked at the news, it was about a patient involved in a murder-suicide. I had treated the gunman.

"The face of gun violence, for me," Fischer said, concluding the story, was "that kid in the back of the car, paralyzed with fear with blood on his clothes."

An ordinary, plain-appearing, blue-eyed white guy from Green Bay, Wisconsin, Fischer has continually thrust himself into areas that are predominantly Black. First in Philadelphia, a city 41% Black and 35% white, and now in Prince George's County, Maryland, a county that is 65% Black and only 19% white. Unlike Gore, a Black man from Brooklyn who attended Morehouse College—one of America's 107 Historically Black Colleges and Universities, Fischer is not who you might anticipate to see at the center of advocacy about the urban gun violence that all too often impacts young men of color. Yet, there he is, shift after shift.

Like me, Fischer no longer searches the newspapers to find news reports about the kind of everyday gun violence he witnesses at work. It is too commonplace to be newsworthy. Yet the slow, steady trickle of handgun crime is how the vast majority of people—typically young and Black or Brown—die by gun violence.

While the young man pulled from the gun-riddled Toyota Corolla recovered in a hospital bed at Hahnemann, he would have had countless hours to lie in bed and reflect on his trauma. Men and women like him, similarly stricken, might allow those initial emotions of fear and anger to coalesce into a plan for revenge. These negative emotions settle into psychological trauma, leading to adjustment disorders—conditions in which we react adversely to negative life experiences. This can persist, triggering lifelong issues such as post-traumatic stress disorder or major depression. For many, channeling these feelings into a desire for peace never arrives. That's precisely the second golden hour of trauma.

***

Not surprisingly, sitting in his hospital room at Memorial Hermann, my neighbor Lee was angry. "Hot as fish grease," he described bluntly. While for many young men, anger might manifest in continued violence, that was unlikely to be the case for Lee. He recalled his nephew, who is now serving time for his involvement in a situation in which one brother killed another, and realized the lesson that for every choice made in life, there are consequences. Recognizing the potential for serious repercussions, Lee dealt with his anger. Today, he harbors no ill will toward his brother.

Another young man, Sherman Spears, lying in hospital bed in Oakland, California, paralyzed from his injuries, decided that instead of engaging in retaliatory violence, he would rather make use of his time to heal other victims of violence. In an interview conducted in 1998, he described the essence of Caught in the Crossfire, a prototypical hospital-based violence intervention program whose inception came about as Sherman lay looking at the tile ceiling of his hospital room.

"When I got shot, there were very few resources to help me deal with my injury on a personal level," Spears told Chela Delgado in a story for the Colorlines website.[10] "I wanted to fill that gap. Crossfire is a response team that goes into the hospital and works with youth, ages 19 and under, who have been recently admitted for violence-related injuries. We counsel the youth and help them set up a life plan so when they leave the hospital they can get connected to resources within their community. But our underlying goal is to talk them into talking to their friends about not seeking retribution for their injuries."

Hospital-based violence intervention programs across this country seek to do exactly that. Their goal is to blunt the psychological trauma of being shot, stabbed, or bludgeoned and transform that energy into something productive. Fischer mentioned Spears's story to me and described violence prevention professionals as the "secret sauce" of hospital-based violence intervention programs across the country. These violence interrupters, as I like to call them, help physicians, nurses, social workers, and policymakers put an end to this public health crisis.

Fischer is currently the policy director for HAVI, the Health Alliance for Violence Intervention. He told me about the organization's mission, one that builds and connects violence intervention programs and promotes equity for victims of violence, as we sat in a quiet corner of the Denver Convention Center looking out on the snowflakes drifting down toward the street below us. Fischer explained that the recipe for successful violence intervention programs requires frontline personnel who can provide victims of violence with longitudinal care, from the moment they arrive in the trauma bay to at least three to six months after their departure from the hospital. These individuals require case management to facilitate their enrollment in community resources as well as peer support from violence interrupters.

Several studies have documented the success of violence intervention programs in the reduction of trauma recidivism, or the recurrence of violence in victims of prior acts. One comparative study in San Francisco demonstrated a 75% reduction in trauma recidivism among patients. Some of the strongest effects were among those who received intensive, early interventions including mental health care, case management, and employment services in the first three months following trauma.[11] Other randomized trials that investigated violence intervention programs saw small reductions among criminal misdemeanor activity,[12] reductions in arrests and convictions for criminal activity,[13] and reductions in self-reported reinjury rates[14] among participants.

Programs like Gore's KAVI and Spears' Crossfire cooperate with HAVI to help end the cycle of violence in this country in ways that have nothing to do with what the NRA would consider gun control. Yet it is still gun violence prevention. It falls on clinicians and communities to work together to stop the cycle of gun violence.

"Recently publicized mass casualty shootings have shown us that we are all vulnerable regardless of where we live," Gore said, "which makes the bystander and the veteran, the teacher and the sibling, the first grader and the gangbanger all equally affected by gun violence. And if they do survive a violent injury, how the consequential posttraumatic stresses diffuse will depend on the immediate treatment the survivors receive."

Neighbors and communities in America can intervene at the local level to reduce the toll of firearm injuries and deaths that pervade our country. Violence intervention programs have demonstrated reductions in repeat trauma and recurrent crime. As I write this, my hospital recently started a violence intervention program to aid in the recovery of the men and women who present to the emergency department for violent injuries.

Physicians play an important role in this epidemic, whether we choose to define violence as harm toward others or harm toward self. I wish the NRA would express an interest in preventing gun violence. One physician I have spoken with thinks that reducing gun violence is the best way to protect the rights of law-abiding gun owners from the what he considers to be the political whims of those who disagree with a broad interpretation of the Second Amendment. But the NRA has abdicated leadership on the issue of preventing gun deaths. Thus, physicians, nurses, social workers, and other health care professionals have pursued this calling for decades. Betz, the red-headed suicide prevention researcher from Denver, rebuts the NRA's claim that physicians consulted no one but themselves when putting forth recommendations about preventing gun violence. "We did consult with you," she tweeted, "but you said you weren't intersted [*sic*] in including suicide prevention topics in your safety courses. Let us know if you change your mind."[15] The NRA hasn't shown interest in supporting violence interrupters either.

"I think we bring a different approach and different solutions," Fischer said, when discussing violence in American communities and the value that health care professionals bring to the table. "Violence affects all of us, just in different ways. When you start thinking about the root of violence being trauma, then all of a sudden there is a central line between all of them. So, you know, the risk of suicide . . . associated with a history of trauma. Homicide . . . trauma. Interpersonal violence . . . trauma. It's the thread that connects all of them. And if we don't address that, it's [to] everyone's detriment."

For the physicians who exclaimed #ThisIsOurLane, a viral hashtag has become a sustaining movement for physician advocacy regarding the epidemic of over 120,000 annual firearm injuries and deaths. Fischer admitted, "I legitimately don't know where public health and medical care starts and stops." There is no clear dividing line for physicians who care about ending gun violence—there are only dashed lines on the pavement that allow them to switch from one lane to the next whenever the need arises to address the issue of gun violence for their patients, their friends and loved ones, and their communities.

"If you believe that violence is a health issue, which I do," Fischer said, "it should be taken care of with patient-centered health-based approaches and public health approaches. Can you imagine any other disease where thousands of people are dying and they say, 'Oh, let's ask the police what to do about that!' It'd be crazy. We don't do that with any other disease." Gun violence isn't simply a law enforcement problem in America; it's a medical problem, it's a mental health problem, it's a public health problem, and it's a problem that physicians, nurses, and others on the health care team are well equipped to solve.

CHAPTER SIXTEEN

We Don't Have to Wait to Act

In 2017, a shooter using 14 different AR-15–style rifles sprayed over 1,000 rounds into the crowd attending the Route 91 Harvest Music Festival in Las Vegas, immediately killing 57 people and injuring over 500.[1] Two years later, ten Democratic presidential candidates assembled in the city that had recently been upended by what is still the deadliest mass shooting in American history. Two physicians who were interviewed for this book—Joseph Sakran and Kyle Fischer—attended the meeting, a Gun Safety Forum in Las Vegas that March for Our Lives and Giffords Courage organized in 2020. The three of us had just coauthored a piece in the blog of the journal *Health Affairs*, the preeminent journal for health policy research, urging physicians to rally behind the concept that had recently motivated health care workers to speak out loudly against the National Rifle Association and to proclaim that #ThisIsOurLane when speaking up on America's endemic gun violence problem.[2] Determined to promote evidence-based health policy, we focused our discussion on potential legislative solutions that the RAND Corporation, the organization the NRA referenced in its misguided tweet suggesting that physicians should "stay in their lane," has found evidence to support.

Because the NRA attempted to discredit the American College of Physicians' 2018 position paper on firearms with the assertion that the authors had incompletely reviewed the data, we had decided to look closer at the source material ourselves.

The NRA wondered "if the [ACP] authors reviewed the evidence, or just found works that suited their needs." Our assessment, ironically enough, was that it was the NRA that had presented nothing more than half-truths, pointing out where the science was inconclusive but ignoring where the science suggested that specific laws might reduce the impact of firearms on injuries and death.

The RAND Corporation's *The Science of Gun Policy* clearly indicated that there were at least six gun laws that the United States should implement now or strengthen in every jurisdiction across this country—universal background checks, minimum age for purchases, child access prevention laws, domestic violence restraining orders (with provisions to remove guns), waiting periods, and permits to purchase. Each would have a proven benefit to save American lives.[3] Additionally, repealing stand-your-ground and concealed carry laws would be equally crucial in tackling America's gun violence epidemic. Voiding these laws could avert deaths that result from rapid escalation of arguments, like what happens in some road rage incidents.

Borrowing a line from the musical *Hamilton*, we penned an opinion piece titled "History Has Its Eye on Us." We focused on evidence-based policies that clinicians should rally around to impact the epidemic of gun violence devastating our communities. Ironically, Alexander Hamilton himself was a victim of gun violence; he died in a duel with Vice President Aaron Burr.[4]

The impetus behind our argument was simple: if the NRA wanted to admonish doctors for overstating the science underlying the RAND Gun Policy Analysis, it shouldn't look at the data selectively. Correcting the NRA's misinformation campaign is one of the major reasons why I set out to write this book. I'm not a gun violence researcher. But I believe that health policy, above all else, should be informed by evidence when that evidence is available. As a physician, I understand the limitations of science. While the best science, at least in the biomedical sphere, usually requires the findings of randomized clinical trials, those types of studies are often not feasible for policy decision-making. In the public health sphere, the next best option is a natural experiment, in which one jurisdiction implements a policy and a similar, nearby jurisdiction does not. Observing the difference between those two locations can shed light on the true impact of policy decisions. *The Science of Gun Policy* typically relies on these types of studies to inform its analysis.

Lower down on the hierarchy of scientific evidence are retrospective studies. These kinds of studies are relatively poor examples from which to draw conclusions pertaining to causality. These studies, either case-control or cross-sectional investigations, have often been used by pro-gun authors to support the concept behind defensive gun use. The RAND Corporation, which the NRA itself has professed is the ideal arbiter of the science, concluded in the 2020 edition of *The Science of Gun Policy* that "rigorous research examining the effects of many state gun policies on officer-involved shootings, *defensive gun use*, hunting and recreation, and the gun industry is virtually nonexistent."[5] Perhaps it is the NRA's own fault, as they were the ones stifling the scientific research that could have shed light on their ideological preferences.

So what are we, as consumers of the evidence and advocates for evidence-based policy, to decide? In the preceding chapters, I have examined *The Science of Gun Policy* and attempted to illustrate how specific laws and regulations might apply through real-life stories—either my own or the stories of colleagues.

The Science of Gun Policy bombards its reader with data—sometimes inconclusive, sometimes weak, sometimes strong—in its assertions about the impacts of various policies that might impact lives in this epidemic of gun violence. Even as I was writing this book, from the first edition of *The Science of Gun Policy* in 2018 to the second edition in 2020, the conclusions about the benefits of some policies—mental health checks, in particular—changed based on an evolving analysis. *The Science of Gun Policy* describes myriad policy levers that our current lawmakers could, and in my opinion should, swiftly implement at the federal, state, and local levels. But you don't have to be a gun violence researcher, an injury prevention specialist, an academic, or even an emergency physician or trauma surgeon to understand the simple steps that will save people's lives. You just have to be willing to be an advocate in your own community.

We don't have to wait to act.

The evidence states that we can save lives through the following policies:

- Background checks through federal firearms licensed dealers for every firearms purchase
- Licenses and permits for individuals who want to buy guns
- Raising the minimum age for all firearm purchases to 21

- Strong child access prevention laws
- Brief waiting periods
- Domestic violence restraining orders that require the relinquishing of existing firearms

States and other jurisdictions that have yet to implement these policies should do so immediately and ensure that their state-based databases, such as court and health care systems, push records into the federal National Instant Criminal Background Check System to combat the epidemic of gun violence in America. Two additional laws should be repealed. Their presence in society should alarm physicians, advocates, and the people who write the laws.

Policy Prescription: Stand-Your-Ground Laws Provide a Rationale for Escalating Conflict toward Violence. Legislators Should Reverse Them

I vividly remember my summer experience as a gangly college student at Brandeis University, where I spent time doing research in Waltham, Massachusetts, a place distinctly different from Atlanta and the South. In the Northeast, people do not have the same penchant for eye contact or saying, "Good morning!" and "Hello!" just because you happen to be passing by on the sidewalk.

One weekend, I walked down from the campus toward the light rail and took the train into Boston. Once inside the subway station, known as "the T" to locals, I sat down next to an older white lady who looked up at me and clutched her purse a little closer. I will always recall that moment as one of the microaggressions that I faced simply because people have been conditioned to view Black men with negative stereotypes. As a young Black man, perhaps I should feel fortunate that a slight gesture based on the color of my skin led only to a brief recoil from an elderly woman. In another situation, perhaps I wouldn't have been so fortunate.

Consider Trayvon Martin, a Black kid who was my height and had a similar build, walking through a neighborhood after purchasing a bag of Skittles and a drink. He was essentially stalked by the captain of the neighborhood watch patrol in a subdivision in the town of Sanford, Florida. Following an altercation, one that a 911 dispatcher urged the overly zealous neighborhood watchman to avoid, Martin lay on the ground, shot dead by a single bullet that traversed his heart and lung.

All of that young man's hopes and dreams of one day becoming an aviator were struck down by a man who would eventually be acquitted of murder because of Florida's stand-your-ground statute that created a culture of approach, provoke, and kill. Stand your ground certainly contributed to the young boy's death.

Every state has some form of this doctrine embedded in common law, something that recognizes that an American man or woman inside their home has the right to defend themselves. But how far does that right travel outside the home? Obviously, if someone approached you attempting to harm you, no one would blame you for defending yourself. But what happens when you initiate the incident and instead of retreating, escalate a situation that never needed to exist in the first place?

The castle doctrine permits a person who is in his or her home to defend it and themselves from harm without any duty to retreat to safety. But a duty to retreat when in public exists in many states. Ohio, Wisconsin, and North Dakota, however, extend the castle doctrine to one's personal vehicle. In some locations, largely in the South, this doctrine extends to any place a person has a legal right to be. Vermont and Washington, DC, remain the only two jurisdictions where a duty to retreat remains supreme.

Florida's statute regarding the castle doctrine is a prototypical bad policy as borne out by the evidence from the RAND Corporation analysis. Stand-your-ground laws clearly increase the risk of total homicides, specifically firearm homicides.

Stand-your-ground laws have no beneficial impacts on other forms of violent crime, suggesting that these laws have not lived up to their purported deterrent effect, as the NRA and other Second Amendment advocates might claim. Lawmakers should repeal stand-your-ground laws, reverting to a more limited use of the castle doctrine to prevent the deaths of their constituents when minor conflicts escalate into public confrontations with deadly consequences.

Policy Prescription: Concealed Carry Laws Should Adhere to the May-Issue Standard

US federal law grants current and retired law enforcement officers the ability to carry firearms in a concealed manner. Even for the average citizen, concealed carry rights are nearly universal, although twenty-three states and the District of Columbia require a permit to do so as of 2023.[6] The other twenty-seven states do not require a permit, and individuals there can simply concealed carry without any form of vetting.

Concealed carry laws differ in several distinct ways, ranging in order of least to most restrictive, from *permitless* carry to *shall-issue* to *may-issue* laws (see fig. 16.1). Among the states that require a permit for someone to carry a concealed weapon, the permitting entity, often law enforcement, must issue it to anyone who meets minimum standards in shall-issue states. In may-issue states, there is some additional leeway for law

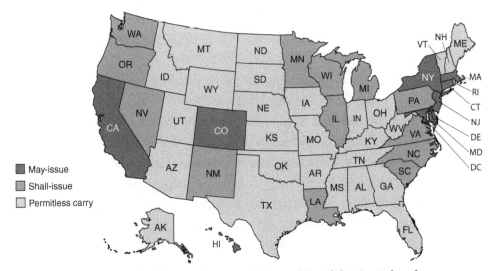

FIGURE 16.1   Concealed Carry Laws. *May-issue (9):* California, Colorado, Connecticut, Delaware, Hawaii, Maryland, Massachusetts, New Jersey, and New York. *Shall-issue (14):* Illinois, Louisiana, Michigan, Minnesota, Nevada, New Mexico, North Carolina, Oregon, Pennsylvania, Rhode Island, South Carolina, Virginia, Washington, and Wisconsin. *Permitless carry (27):* Alabama, Alaska, Arizona, Arkansas, Florida, Georgia, Idaho, Indiana, Iowa, Kansas, Kentucky, Maine, Mississippi, Missouri, Montana, Nebraska, New Hampshire, North Dakota, Ohio, Oklahoma, South Dakota, Tennessee, Texas, Utah, Vermont, West Virginia, and Wyoming.

Source: https://giffords.org/lawcenter/gun-laws/browse-state-gun-laws/?filter 0=,281. (January 2024)

enforcement to prevent issuing a permit to people who might be a threat to themselves or others, even if they otherwise would be eligible by virtue of the fact that they are not a felon, are not subject to a mental health restriction, or are not a convicted domestic abuser.

Shouldn't a small-town sheriff who knows his community well have some discretion when reviewing applications from people in the town for concealed carry licenses? What if there was a violent man in that community who has been drinking when he walks through the door and who, in anger, strikes his wife repeatedly, but each time the cops come out for a domestic disturbance they are told that she simply fell down the stairs? What would happen if that man applied for a concealed carry license? In a shall-issue state, the man would easily receive it; the cops would be obliged to give the man his permit. In a may-issue state, the sheriff who suspects domestic violence but has not yet proven it in a court of law might wisely reject the application and potentially save the life of that man's wife.

Lonny Pulkrabek, a Jefferson County sheriff who laments that his state legislature voted to make Iowa a shall-issue state in 2011, no longer has any discretion when issuing a concealed carry permit. He reported that in 2018, "I've already got 140 people through May that have criminal records that have permits, that were issued permits to carry. We've seen a lot more people with lengthy criminal histories who in fact are willing to go through and jump through the hoops and get the permit to carry it legally. And you know the problem with that is, is you know when they said 'Criminals were already carrying,' well back then criminals were carrying, but if they got caught carrying there were consequences. And now criminals are carrying and they're carrying legally."[7]

Sheriff Pulkrabek maintains a "wall of shame" of the several hundred concealed carry permits he has been forced to issue to Iowans with criminal records because the state elected to follow an inferior law over a decade ago. Researchers, utilizing the natural experiment set by the various policies in force in different states, have detected differences between states with divergent legal frameworks as they pertain to concealed carry. *The Science of Gun Policy* indicates that shall-issue laws, such as Iowa's, may increase overall violent crime compared to may-

issue laws.[8] Based on the underlying research, scientists estimate that in ten years following a transition to the more
permissive type of concealed carry law, violent crime increases
by up to 15%. How much worse might the situation be in states
that exercise permitless carry? As a matter of scientific fact, I
honestly cannot answer that question, but as a public health
expert, prudence dictates that I should focus on convincing the
states with permitless carry policies to adopt some form of
concealed carry permitting and to improve the vetting process
from shall-issue to may-issue in the states with the weaker ver-
sion of the law. Since concealed carry laws have been shown to
increase violent crime, shouldn't we have some say about who
walks around town with a hidden firearm? Unfortunately,
many state legislatures haven't been following the science.
Iowa recently went even farther afield, along with Tennessee
and Texas, by weakening their laws to allow for permitless
carry beginning in the summer of 2021. I worry that it will
lead to more crime and more bloodshed.

- Stand-your-ground laws clearly increase the risk of
  total homicides and specifically firearm homicides.
- Shall-issue concealed-carry laws increase overall
  violent crime compared to may-issue laws.

Epilogue

The controversies over measures as simple as wearing a mask during the COVID-19 pandemic demonstrate the difficulties facing physicians and public health professionals focused on evidence-based solutions to our nation's most pressing public health challenges, especially when they regard politically charged issues such as gun violence prevention. A challenge recognized nearly 50 years ago, subsequently stifled by the enemies of science for two and a half decades, the epidemic of gun violence continues to burn through American communities at an ever-increasing pace. From 1990 to 2021, over 1.1 million Americans lost their lives to firearms.[1] While writing this book, however, some progress has been made.

Congress approved $25 million for fiscal year 2020 specifically to fund gun violence research at the CDC and the NIH. This was the first time since the Dickey Amendment, which has starved the injury prevention community of funding and threatened the careers of injury prevention researchers, that federal funding prioritized looking into firearms as a vector for death and disability. While funding has finally started to flow, it comes at a huge deficit compared with what the research community deserves for a condition with death rates as severe as motor vehicle crashes. Firearm injury prevention receives a small fraction of federal dollars relative to the amount we spend studying other causes of morbidity and mortality.[2]

The Bipartisan Safer Communities Act, signed into law by President Biden in 2022, provided grants to states to create emergency risk protection orders, closed the "boyfriend loophole," and provided $250 million to support community violence intervention initiatives.

Yet there is so much more that should be done. It falls on us to decide whether to listen to science or continue to be scammed by agents of chaos such as the NRA. As Art Kellermann told me regarding his past work, he was not trying to tell anyone what to do regarding their personal decision to own firearms, he was merely trying to provide people with information and a true discussion of risk so they could make an educated decision for themselves.

The COVID-19 pandemic spread across the world with a ferocity unbeknownst to any but the oldest of us who remember the influenza pandemic of 1918. In this pandemic, the average American learned what public health can and cannot do. We've witnessed the scientific method unfold before our eyes as we waited for vaccines and treatments to be created in record time. Just as public health measures such as staying at home in the early phases of the COVID crisis, wearing masks once society began to open, and vaccination tamed this most recent pandemic, I have faith that science can do the same thing for endemic gun violence in America.

The science compiled by the RAND Corporation suggests a series of potential legislative approaches that will save the lives of some of the over 45,000 Americans who die by firearms each year. We should not be mistaken into thinking that we can eliminate every injury, every death, or every shooting, but we must recognize that we can positively impact our fellow Americans, save lives, and relieve suffering by implementing some very simple laws that I describe in this book. After I submitted the earlier draft of this book to the publisher, a third edition of *The Science of Gun Policy* was released in 2022. Fortunately, it reinforced the policies I advocate for in this book. But it also added two new ones due to evolving evidence. It is now understood that private background checks *can* cut the number of firearm homicides and that bans on high-capacity magazines *can* reduce the number and lethality of mass shootings.

Community countermeasures such as violence intervention programs to prevent interpersonal violence and gun buddies to stall self-directed violence may also work but still require additional, rigorous research studies to back them up.

As clinicians we know the facts, but it is our stories that truly matter. In the trauma bay, in the emergency department, in the operating room, in the rehabilitation center, and in every single clinic visit, health care workers must place the human narrative back into the lifeless statistics around gun violence. If we as health professionals are to deliver on the shared hope, that we can stop disease before it occurs, we must fervently believe that dealing with gun violence is part of our job description not just at the beside but also in our interactions with society.

Firearms represent just one vector for the diseases of depression, hostility, and hate—all of which can be summed up under the term violence. They transmit injuries and death to over 120,000 Americans every year. Those of us who witness the human toll of this uniquely American epidemic, must rise to the challenge of speaking this truth to our patients, to our communities, and to those with the power to affect change.

The NRA will always try to silence us. Nevertheless, doctors, nurses, and health care workers must remember and be unafraid to boldly proclaim:

THIS.

IS.

OUR.

LANE.

NOTES

Prologue

1. JRA (with acknowledgements to Siân Anis). Virchow misquoted, part-quoted, and the real McCoy. *J Epidemiol Community Health.* 2006 Aug;60(8):671.

2. Rudolf Virchow on Pathology Education, http://www.pathguy.com /virchow.htm.

1. Trauma

1. Kochanek KD, Murphy SL, Xu JQ, Arias E. Deaths: Final data for 2020. *National Vital Statistics Reports.* 2023;72(10). Hyattsville, MD: National Center for Health Statistics.

2. Follman M, Lurie J, Lee J, et al. The true cost of gun violence in America. *Mother Jones.* April 15, 2015. https://www.motherjones .com/politics/2015/04/true-cost-of-gun-violence-in-america/.

3. Rees CA, Monuteaux MC, Steidley I, et al. Trends and disparities in firearm fatalities in the United States, 1990–2021. *JAMA Netw Open.* 2022;5(11):e2244221.

4. Karp A. Estimating global civilian held firearms numbers. June 2018. Small Arms Survey. http://www.smallarmssurvey.org /fileadmin/docs/T-Briefing-Papers/SAS-BP-Civilian-Firearms -Numbers.pdf.

5. Kalesan B, Vyliparambil MA, Zuo Y, et al. Cross-sectional study of loss of life expectancy at different ages related to firearm deaths among black and white Americans. *BMJ Evidence-Based Medicine.* 2019;24:55–58.

2. Contagion

1. Moritsugu K. Chinese doctor who sounded the alarm about the virus dies. Associated Press. February 6, 2020.

2. He warned of coronavirus. Here's what he told us before he died. *New York Times*. February 7, 2020.

3. Scutti S. Measles rarely kills in the US—but when it does, here's how. *CNN*. February 5, 2019. https://www.cnn.com/2019/02/05 /health/how-measles-kills-explainer/index.html.

4. Thomas JD. Accidents don't happen. *Emory Magazine*. Summer 1995. https://www.emory.edu/EMORY_MAGAZINE/summer95 /kellermann.html.

5. Rosenberg T. Fighting street gun violence as if it were a contagion. *New York Times*. May 8, 2018.

6. Ransford C, Decker RB, and Slutkin G. *Cure Violence*. Report on the Cure Violence model adaptation in San Pedro Sula, Honduras. November 2016.

7. World Health Organization. Malaria. April 1, 2021. https://www .who.int/news-room/fact-sheets/detail/malaria.

8. Butts JA, Roman CG, Bostwick L, et al. Cure violence: A public health model to reduce gun violence. *Annu Rev Public Health*. 2015;36(Mar 18):39–53.

3. What's Going On?

1. Kellermann AL, Reay DT. Protection or peril? An analysis of firearm-related deaths in the home. *N Engl J Med*. 1986;314 (24):1557–1560.

2. Sommers BD, Long SK, Baicker K. Changes in mortality after Massachusetts health care reform: a quasi-experimental study. *Ann Intern Med*. 2014;160 (9):585–593.

4. The Revolt against Science

1. United States. Congress. House Committee on Ways and Means. *National Firearms Act. Hearings: Seventy-third Congress, Second session, on H.R. 9066*. U.S. Government Printing Office, 1934.

2. Suess J. NRA: "Revolt at Cincinnati" molded National Rifle Association. *Cincinnati Enquirer*. March 8, 2018. https://www .cincinnati.com/story/news/politics/2018/03/08/revolt-cincinnati

-molded-nra-did-you-know-jeff-suess-schism-within-national-rifle
-association-led/404628002/.

3. A brief history of the NRA. NRA.org. https://home.nra.org/about
-the-nra/.

4. Sanson LJ. History of a case in which excision of a portion of the
lower jaw was practised by M. Dupuytren, to obtain the re-union of
fragments of this bone, resulting from a fracture of it with loss of
substance and want of consolidation, consequent on a wound by a
fire-arm. *Lond Med Phys J.* 1820 Sep;44(259):197–205.

5. Maiming by firearms, etc. *The Hospital.* 1888 Aug 11;4 (98):306.

6. On wounds from fire-arms without ball. *Buffalo Med J Mon Rev
Med Surg Sci.* 1847; 2(11):668–670.

7. As of January 2020, 7,981 publications in the PubMed database
contained the word *firearm*. Limiting the search to studies on
humans in the English language yields 5,883 publications dating
as far back as the nineteenth century. There were 3 articles in the
1920s, 13 in the 1940s, and 58 in the 1950s.

8. Rushforth NB, Ford AB, Hirsch CS, et al. Violent death in a
metropolitan county. Changing patterns in homicide (1958–74).
N Engl J Med. 1977 Sep 8;297(10):531–538.

9. I would like to thank the anonymous reviewers of this book who
suggested mentioning several physicians who should be credited
with laying the public health foundation upon which the many
other physicians mentioned in this book have built their advocacy
careers: Steve Hargarten, a professor of emergency medicine and
founding director of the Comprehensive Injury Center at the
Medical College of Wisconsin; Frederick P. Rivara, a professor of
pediatrics and epidemiology at the University of Washington at
Seattle Children's Hospital; and Carnell Cooper, the chief medical
officer of Northeast Methodist Hospital, who as a surgeon created
the violence intervention program at the R Adams Cowley Shock
Trauma Center at the University of Maryland. Although this book
focuses solely on physician-advocates, readers should realize that
this work has been supported by the tireless and sometimes
dangerous efforts from nurses such as Therese S. Richmond, the

Andrea B. Laporte Professor of Nursing and Associate Dean for Research & Innovation at the University of Pennsylvania; epidemiologists such as Charlie Branas, the chair of the department of epidemiology at the Columbia University Mailman School of Public Health; economists such as David Hemenway, a professor of health policy at the Harvard T.H. Chan School of Public Health, director of the Harvard Injury Control Research Center, and author of the book *Private Guns, Public Health*; and Daniel W. Webster the Bloomberg Professor of American Health at the Johns Hopkins Bloomberg School of Public Health and director of the Center for Gun Policy and Research at Johns Hopkins University.

10. Brent DA, Perper JA, Goldstein CE, et al. Risk factors for adolescent suicide. A comparison of adolescent suicide victims with suicidal inpatients. *Arch Gen Psychiatry*. 1988 Jun;45(6):581–588.

11. Brent DA, Perper JA, Moritz G, et al. Firearms and adolescent suicide. A community case-control study. *Am J Dis Child*. 1993 Oct;147(10):1066–1071.

12. Brent DA, Perper J, Moritz G, et al. Suicide in adolescents with no apparent psychopathology. *J Am Acad Child Adolesc Psychiatry*. 1993 May;32(3):494–500.

13. Conner A, Azrael D, Miller M. Suicide case-fatality rates in the United States, 2007 to 2014: A nationwide population-based study. *Ann Intern Med*. 2019 Dec 17;171(12):885–895.

14. Wintemute GJ, Teret SP, Kraus JF. The epidemiology of firearm deaths among residents of California. *West J Med*. 1987 Mar;146(3): 374–377.

15. *Am J Health Promot*. 1992 Jul–Aug;6(6):451–464.

16. *Health Aff (Millwood)*. 1993 Winter;12(4):198–208.

17. Kellermann AL, Rivara FP. Silencing the science on gun research. *JAMA*. 2013 Feb 13;309(6):549–550.

18. Kellermann AL. Comment: Gunsmoke—changing public attitudes toward smoking and firearms. *Am J Public Health*. 1997 Jun;87(6): 910–913.

19. Thompson M. Thompson: Former rep. Jay Dickey calls to end federal ban on gun violence research. Press release. https://

mikethompson.house.gov/newsroom/press-releases/thompson
-former-rep-jay-dickey-calls-end-federal-ban-gun-violence
-research.

5. Canary in the Coal Mine

1. WHO. Violence against women. March 9, 2021. https://www.who
.int/news-room/fact-sheets/detail/violence-against-women.

2. Campbell JC, Webster D, Koziol-McLain J, et al. Risk factors for
femicide in abusive relationships: Results from a multisite case
control study. *Am J Public Health*. 2003 Jul;93(7):1089–1097.

3. JRA (with acknowledgements to Siân Anis). Virchow misquoted,
part-quoted, and the real McCoy. *J Epidemiol Community Health*.
2006 Aug;60(8):671.

4. Ndungu N. Legislating against sexual violence in Kenya: An
interview with the Hon. Njoki Ndungu. *Reprod Health Matters*.
2007 May;15(29):149–154.

5. Branas CC, Richmond TS, Culhane DP, et al. Investigating the link
between gun possession and gun assault. *Am J Public Health*.
2009 Nov;99(11):2034–2040.

6. Jamieson C. Gun violence research: History of the federal funding
freeze. American Psychological Association. February 2013.
https://www.apa.org/science/about/psa/2013/02/gun-violence (site
discontinued).

7. Schneider C, Suggs E. CDC: Politics affected gun violence research.
Atlanta Journal Constitution. December 19, 2012. https://www.ajc
.com/news/cdc-politics-affected-gun-violence-research/H1aKOO
51fbkfMLOehRnyrK/.

8. Sandy Hook Elementary School shooting. https://en.wikipedia.org
/wiki/Sandy_Hook_Elementary_School_shooting.

9. President Obama makes a statement on the shooting in Newtown,
Connecticut, December 14, 2012. https://web.archive.org/web
/20130815010511/http://www.whitehouse.gov/photos-and-video
/video/2012/12/14/president-obama-makes-statement-shooting
-newtown-connecticut#transcript.

6. This Is Our Lane

1. Butkus R, Doherty R, Bornstein SS, et al. Reducing firearm injuries and deaths in the United States: A position paper from the American College of Physicians. *Ann Intern Med.* 2018 Nov 20;169(10):704–707.

2. Lowes R. Appeals court overturns Florida's physician "gun-gag" law. Medscape. February 16, 2017. https://www.medscape.com/viewarticle/875942.

3. Weinberger SE, Hoyt DB, Lawrence HC 3rd, et al. Firearm-related injury and death in the United States: A call to action from 8 health professional organizations and the American Bar Association. *Ann Intern Med.* 2015 Apr 7;162(7):513–516.

4. National Rifle Association. Twitter Post. November 7, 2018. 1:43 P.M. https://twitter.com/nra/status/1060256567914909702.

5. Gonzalez M. Twitter Post. November 7, 2018. 9:10 P.M. https://twitter.com/Zindoctor/status/1060338793847418885.

6. Ranney M. Twitter Post. November 7, 2018. 6:41 P.M. https://twitter.com/meganranney/status/1060301303644078081.

7. The following individuals contributed materially to our op-ed piece: N. Seth Trueger, MD, MPH; Bích-Mây Nguyễn, MD, MPH; Orlando Sola, MD, MPH; Elizabeth DuPre, MD; and Esther Choo, MD, MPH.

8. Dark C, Fischer K, and Ranney M. Docs to NRA: Gun violence is in our lane. *Houston Chronicle.* November 12, 2018. https://www.houstonchronicle.com/opinion/outlook/article/Docs-to-NRA-Gun-violence-is-in-our-lane-Opinion-13385277.php.

9. Matthews G. Twitter Post. November 4, 2019. 6:06 P.M. https://twitter.com/chimoose/status/1191506958383222784?s=20.

10. Schuur JD, Decker H, Baker O. Association of physician organization-affiliated political action committee contributions with US House of Representatives and Senate candidates' stances on firearm regulation. *JAMA Netw Open.* 2019 Feb 1;2(2):e187831.

7. Rationally Irrational

1. MD magazine poll on curbing gun violence finds most doctors have guns. Press release. HCP Live. January 25, 2016. https://www .hcplive.com/view/md-magazine-poll-on-curbing-gun-violence -finds-most-doctors-have-guns; Becher EC, Cassel CK, Nelson EA. Physician firearm ownership as a predictor of firearm injury prevention practice. *Am J Public Health*. 2000 Oct;90(10): 1626–1628.

2. Farcy DA, Doria N, Moreno-Walton L, et al. Emergency physician survey on firearm injury prevention: Where can we improve? *West J Emerg Med*. 2021 Feb 8;22(2):257–265.

3. Frank E, Kellerman A. Firearm ownership among female physicians in the United States. *South Med J*. 1999 Nov;92(11): 1083–1088.

4. Frank E, Carrera JS, Prystowsky J, et al. Firearm-related personal and clinical characteristics of US medical students. *South Med J*. 2006 Mar;99(3):216–225.

5. Parker K, Menasce Horowitz J, Igielnik R, et al. America's complex relationship with guns. Pew Research Center. June 22, 2017. https://www.pewresearch.org/social-trends/2017/06/22/americas -complex-relationship-with-guns/.

6. Mesic A, Franklin L, Cansever A, et al. The relationship between structural racism and Black-white disparities in fatal police shootings at the state level. *J Natl Med Assoc*. 2018;110(2):106–116.

7. Juzwiak R, Chan A. Unarmed people of color killed by police, 1999–2014. Gawker. December 8, 2014. https://gawker.com /unarmed-people-of-color-killed-by-police-1999-2014-1666672349 (site discontinued).

8. For more on Dr. Brian H. Williams's story of the 2016 Dallas police ambush, read Yasmin S. Black doctor who treated Dallas shooting victims speaks honestly about supporting and fearing police. *Dallas Morning News*. July 11, 2016. https://www.dallasnews.com /news/2016/07/11/black-doctor-who-treated-dallas-shooting -victims-speaks-honestly-about-supporting-and-fearing-police/.

9. McClellan C, Tekin E. Stand Your Ground laws, homicides, and injuries. *J. Hum. Res.* 2017; 52(3):621–653; Stand Your Ground. Giffords Law Center to Prevent Gun Violence. 2023. https://lawcenter.giffords.org/gun-laws/policy-areas/guns-in-public/stand-your-ground-laws/#state.

10. Degli Esposti M, Wiebe DJ, Gasparrini A, et al. Analysis of "Stand Your Ground" self-defense laws and statewide rates of homicides and firearm homicides. *JAMA Netw Open.* 2022;5(2):e220077.

8. A Well-Regulated Militia

1. Rhee PM, Acosta J, Bridgeman A, et al. Survival after emergency department thoracotomy: Review of published data from the past 25 years. *J Am Coll Surg.* 2000;190(3):288–298. doi:10.1016/s1072-7515(99)00233-1.

2. Kochanek KD, Murphy SL, Xu JQ, Arias E. Deaths: Final data for 2020. *National Vital Statistics Reports.* 2023;72(10). Hyattsville, MD: National Center for Health Statistics.

3. Leap E. I'm a physician and a gun owner. MedPageToday. September 11, 2018. https://www.medpagetoday.com/opinion/kevinmd/75033.

4. Eaton, WJ. Ford, Carter, Reagan push for gun ban. *Los Angeles Times.* May 5, 1994. https://www.latimes.com/archives/la-xpm-1994-05-05-mn-54185-story.html.

5. Gun ownership figures revealed 25 years on from Port Arthur massacre. The University of Sydney. April 28, 2021. https://www.sydney.edu.au/news-opinion/news/2021/04/28/new-gun-ownership-figures-revealed-25-years-on-from-port-arthur.html.

6. Morral AR, Ramchand R, Smart R, et al. *The Science of Gun Policy: A Critical Synthesis of Research Evidence on the Effects of U.S. Gun Policies.* RAND Corporation; 2020. The jurisdictions that have banned assault weapons are California, Connecticut, Hawaii, Maryland, Massachusetts, New Jersey, New York, and the District of Columbia.

7. Cox JW. *Children under Fire.* Harper Collins; 2021.

8. Miller M, Hepburn L, Azrael D. Firearm acquisition without background checks: Results of a national survey. *Ann Intern Med.* 2017;166(4):233–239.

9. An Ounce of Prevention

1. The assassination attempt on Ronald Reagan, 30 Years On. *PBS Newshour.* March 3, 2011. https://www.pbs.org/video/pbs -newshour-the-assassination-attempt-on-ronald-reagan -30-years-on/.

2. Ronald Reagan's close call. *CBS News.* YouTube video. March 27, 2011. https://www.youtube.com/watch?v=XGWqaG817pA.

3. Guns. Gallup. 2023. https://news.gallup.com/poll/1645 /guns.aspx.

4. National Instant Criminal Background Check System (NICS). Federal Bureau of Investigations. Accessed: April 18, 2022. https://www.fbi.gov/services/cjis/nics.

5. Quora contributor. What would happen if we eliminated the world's mosquitoes? Forbes. September 13, 2017. https://www .forbes.com/sites/quora/2017/09/13/what-would-happen-if-we -eliminated-the-worlds-mosquitoes/#4838a0bd11f6.

6. Chapman S, Alpers P, Jones M. Association between gun law reforms and intentional firearm deaths in Australia, 1979–2013. *JAMA.* 2016 Jul 19;316(3):291–299.

7. Gun Violence Archive. https://www.gunviolencearchive.org; Silverstein J. There were more mass shootings than days in 2019. *CBS News.* January 2, 2019. https://www.cbsnews.com/news/mass -shootings-2019-more-than-days-365/.

8. Kaufman EJ, Wiebe DJ, Xiong RA, et al. Epidemiologic trends in fatal and nonfatal firearm injuries in the US, 2009–2017. *JAMA Intern Med.* 2021;181(2):237–244.

9. Miller M, Hepburn L, Azrael D. Firearm acquisition without background checks: Results of a national survey. *Ann Intern Med.* 2017;166(4):233–239.

10. A Pound of Cure

1.   Gani F, Sakran JV, Canner JK. Emergency department visits for firearm-related injuries in the United States, 2006–14. *Health Aff (Millwood)*. 2017;36(10):1729–1738.

2.   Haddon W Jr. Advances in the epidemiology of injuries as a basis for public policy. *Public Health Rep*. 1980;95(5):411–421.

3.   Dolak K. Gun debate spurred by Kennedy assassination rages on today. *ABC News*. November 20, 2013. https://abcnews.go.com/US /gun-debate-spurred-kennedy-assassination-rages-today/story?id =20677433.

4.   Dickenson M. Bush's assassination of the Brady Bill. *Washington Post*. November 2, 1992. https://www.washingtonpost.com/archive /opinions/1992/11/02/bushs-assassination-of-the-brady-bill /ed6ec050-fda2-4d5e-b886-99fc445da84a/.

5.   US Department of Justice. Federal Bureau of Investigation. Criminal Justice Information Services Division. National Instant Criminal Background Check System (NICS) Section. *2019 Operations Report*. https://www.fbi.gov/file-repository/2019-nics -operations-report.pdf/view.

6.   Giffords Law Center. Universal Background Checks. Accessed July 2, 2020. https://lawcenter.giffords.org/gun-laws/policy-areas /background-checks/universal-background-checks/#state. California, Colorado, Connecticut, Delaware, Maryland, Nevada, New Jersey, New Mexico, New York, Oregon, Pennsylvania, Rhode Island, Vermont, Virginia, Washington, and the District of Columbia.

7.   Bowes M. Va.'s new universal background check law, set to begin Wednesday, centers on private sales of firearms. *Richmond Times Dispatch*. June 30, 2020. https://richmond.com/news/virginia/va-s -new-universal-background-check-law-set-to-begin-wednesday -centers-on-private-sales/article_297ecf96-abd5-51d8-bd79 -a4bb19c6248c.html.

8.   Miller M, Hepburn L, Azrael D. Firearm acquisition without background checks: Results of a national survey. *Ann Intern Med*. 2017;166:233–239.

9. Wang, J. Guns are often obtained just days before a crime, study finds. *UChicago News*. June 18, 2019. https://news.uchicago.edu /story/guns-are-often-obtained-just-days-crime-study-finds.

10. Morral AR, Ramchand R, Smart R, et al. *The Science of Gun Policy: A Critical Synthesis of Research Evidence on the Effects of U.S. Gun Policies*. RAND Corporation; 2020, 123–147.

11. National Instant Criminal Background Check System celebrates 20 years of service. *CJIS Link*. November 30, 2018. https://le.fbi .gov/cjis-division/cjis-link/national-instant-criminal-background -check-system-celebrates-20-years-of-service.

12. Criminal Justice Information Services Division, National Instant Criminal Background Check System (NICS) Section. *2018 Operations Report*. https://www.fbi.gov/file-repository/2018-nics -operations-report.pdf/view.

13. Knapp A. FBI had resources to halt Dylann Roof's gun buy, but it didn't use them—and still doesn't. *Post and Courier* (Charleston, SC). February 4, 2018. https://www.postandcourier.com/church _shooting/fbi-had-resources-to-halt-dylann-roofs-gun-buy-but -it-didnt-use-them-and/article_452b95ea-0705-11e8-8bc9-8723f 84ce9dd.html.

14. Adomaitis G. Berlin murder victim told neighbor about gun permit application, then nothing. NJ.com. June 5, 2015. https://www.nj .com/camden/2015/06/berlin_murder_victim_told_neighbor _about_gun_permi.html.

15. Morral et al. *The Science of Gun Policy*, 167–183.

16. Cobler N. Cornyn's gun background check bill works, report says. *Austin American Statesman*. November 27, 2019.

17. Butkus R, Doherty R, Bornstein SS, et al. Reducing firearm injuries and deaths in the United States: A position paper from the American College of Physicians. *Ann Intern Med*. 2018;169(10):704–707; Talley CL, Campbell BT, Jenkins DH, et al. Recommendations from the American College of Surgeons Committee on Trauma's Firearm Strategy Team (FAST) workgroup: Chicago consensus I. *J Am Coll Surg*. 2019;228(2):198–206.

18. Manchester J. Poll: 97 percent support background checks for all gun buyers. *The Hill.* February 20, 2018.

19. Dark C, Sakran JV, Fischer K. History has its eye on us: Clinicians should rally behind "This Is Our Lane." February 21, 2019. *Health Affairs Forefront.* https://www.healthaffairs.org/content/forefront /history-has-its-eye-us-clinicians-should-rally-behind-our-lane.

11. The Mental Health Paradox

1. Dark C. Catching up with ACEP president Dr. Chris Kang. *ACEP Now.* 41(12):1, 9–10.

2. Patel B, Vilendrer S, Kling SMR, et al. Using a real-time locating system to evaluate the impact of telemedicine in an emergency department during COVID-19: Observational study. *J Med Internet Res.* 2021 26;23(7):e29240.

3. Conner A, Azrael D, Miller M. Suicide Case-fatality rates in the United States, 2007 to 2014: A nationwide population-based study. *Ann Intern Med.* 2019 Dec 17;171(12):885–895.

4. National Alliance on Mental Illness. Mental health conditions. https://www.nami.org/learn-more/mental-health-conditions.

5. Morral AR, Ramchand R, Smart R, et al. *The Science of Gun Policy: A Critical Synthesis of Research Evidence on the Effects of U.S. Gun Policies.* RAND Corporation; 2020, 123–147.

6. Grinshteyn E, Hemenway D. Violent death rates: The U.S. compared with other high-income OECD countries, 2010. *Am J Med.* 2016;129(3): 266–273; Richardson EG, Hemenway D. Homicide, suicide, and unintentional firearm fatality; comparing the United States with other high-income countries. *J. Trauma* 2011;70(1):238–243.

7. Louisiana, Alabama, and Alaska had the highest rates of firearm mortality in the country in 2016 (21.3 to 23.3 per 100,000). Firearm Mortality by State. CDC. National Center for Health Statistics. March 1, 2022. https://www.cdc.gov/nchs/pressroom /sosmap/firearm_mortality/firearm.htm.

8. When I originally wrote this testimony, firearms were the number two killer of children in the United States; by 2020, they were the

number one cause of death for kids. See Johns Hopkins Center for Gun Violence Solutions. *A Year in Review: 2020 Gun Deaths in the U.S.* Johns Hopkins Center for Gun Violence Solutions; 2022. https://publichealth.jhu.edu/gun-violence-solutions.

9. Dark C. Leadership and professional development: Never gets easy. *J Hosp Med.* 2023 Sept. https://pubmed.ncbi.nlm.nih.gov/37700513/. Epub ahead of print.

10. Kochanek KD, Murphy SL, Xu JQ, Arias E. Deaths: Final data for 2020. *National Vital Statistics Reports.* 2023;72(10). Hyattsville, MD: National Center for Health Statistics.

11. ESFGV. Prevent firearm suicide: Colorado. https://preventfire armsuicide.efsgv.org/states/colorado/#:~:text=Suicides%20make %20up%2077%25%20of%20all%20firearm%20deaths,Colorado %2C%20including%2037%20children%20and%20teens%20%280 -19%20years%29.

12. Wintemute GJ, Parham CA, Beaumont JJ, et al. Mortality among recent purchasers of handguns. *N Engl J Med.* 1999;341(21): 1583–1589.

13. Betz E. How to talk about guns and suicide. YouTube video. https://www.youtube.com/watch?v=PwBgcjDVxxE.

14. Deisenhammer EA, Ing CM, Strauss R, et al. The duration of the suicidal process: How much time is left for intervention between consideration and accomplishment of a suicide attempt? *J Clin Psychiatry.* 2009;70(1):19–24.

15. Miller IW, Camargo CA Jr, Arias SA, et al. Suicide prevention in an emergency department population: The ED-SAFE study. *JAMA Psychiatry.* 2017;74(6):563–570.

16. Owens D, Horrocks J, House A. Fatal and non-fatal repetition of self-harm. Systematic review. *Br J Psychiatry.* 2002;181:193–199.

17. Spicer RS, Miller TR. Suicide acts in 8 states: Incidence and case fatality rates by demographics and method. *Am J Public Health.* 2000;90:1885–1891; Miller M, Azrael D, Hemenway D. The epidemiology of case fatality rates for suicide in the Northeast. *Ann Emerg Med.* 2004;43:723–730; Conner A, Azrael D, Miller M. Suicide case-fatality rates in the United States, 2007 to 2014: A

nationwide population-based study. *Ann Intern Med.* 2019;171(12): 885-895.

18. Gunnell D, Fernando R, Hewagama M, et al. The impact of pesticide regulations on suicide in Sri Lanka. *Int J Epidemiol.* 2007;36(6):1235-1242.

19. Kreitman N. The coal gas story. United Kingdom suicide rates, 1960-71. *Br J Prev Soc Med.* 1976;30(2):86-93; Hawton K. United Kingdom legislation on pack sizes of analgesics: Background, rationale, and effects on suicide and deliberate self-harm. *Suicide Life Threat Behav.* 2002;32(3):223-229.

20. Johnson RM, Coyne-Beasley T. Lethal means reduction: What have we learned? *Curr Opin Pediatr.* 2009;21(5):635-640.

21. Morral et al. *The Science of Gun Policy*, 167-187.

22. Morral et al. *The Science of Gun Policy*.

12. Think of the Children

1. McCarthy A. Child access prevention laws spare gun deaths in children. Boston Children's Hospital. March 2, 2020. https://answers.childrenshospital.org/child-access-prevention-laws-spare-gun-deaths-in-children/.

2. Azad HA, Monuteaux MC, Rees CA, et al. Child access prevention firearm laws and firearm fatalities among children aged 0 to 14 years, 1991-2016. *JAMA Pediatr.* 2020;174(5):463-469.

3. CDC. National Center for Health Statistics. Homicide mortality by state. March 2, 2022. https://www.cdc.gov/nchs/pressroom/sosmap/homicide_mortality/homicide.htm.

4. CDC. National Center for Health Statistics. Suicide mortality by state. March 1, 2022. https://www.cdc.gov/nchs/pressroom/sosmap/suicide-mortality/suicide.htm.

5. Goldstick JE, Cunningham RM, Carter PM. Current causes of death in children and adolescents in the United States. *N Engl J Med.* 2022;386(20):1955-1956.

6. Arain M, Haque M, Johal L, et al. Maturation of the adolescent brain. *Neuropsychiatr Dis Treat.* 2013;9:449-461. https://doi.org/10.2147/NDT.S39776.

7. H.R. 717. Raise the Age Act. 116th Congress. Congress.gov. https://www.congress.gov/bill/116th-congress/house-bill/717?q=%7B%22se arch%22%3A%5B%22Raise+the+Age+Act%22%5D%7D&s=2&r=1.

8. Kellermann AL, Reay DT. Protection or peril? An analysis of firearm-related deaths in the home. *N Engl J Med*. 1986;314 (24):1557–1560. doi:10.1056/NEJM198606123142406.

9. Azrael D, Cohen J, Salhi C, et al. Firearm storage in gun-owning households with children: Results of a 2015 national survey. *J Urban Health*. 2018;95(3):295–304. doi:10.1007/s11524-018 -0261-7

10. Giffords Law Center. Child access prevention. https://giffords.org /lawcenter/gun-laws/policy-areas/child-consumer-safety/child -access-prevention/.

11. Monuteaux MC, Azrael D, Miller M. Association of increased safe household firearm storage with firearm suicide and unintentional death among us youths. *JAMA Pediatr*. 2019;173(7):657–662. doi:10.1001/jamapediatrics.2019.1078.

12. Hamilton EC, Miller CC 3rd, Cox CS Jr, et al. Variability of child access prevention laws and pediatric firearm injuries. *J Trauma Acute Care Surg*. 2018;84(4):613–619. doi:10.1097/TA.000000000 0001786.

13. Morral AR, Ramchand R, Smart R, et al. *The Science of Gun Policy: A Critical Synthesis of Research Evidence on the Effects of U.S. Gun Policies*. RAND Corporation; 2020, 251–275.

14. H.R. 4062. Blair Holt Firearm Owner Licensing and Record of Sale Act of 2019. 116th Congress. https://www.congress.gov/bill /116th-congress/house-bill/4062/actions?r=17&s=1.

13. Under the Gun

1. Jeltsen M. Tamara O'Neal was almost erased from the story of her own murder. *Huffington Post*. November 21, 2018. https://www .huffpost.com/entry/tamara-oneal-chicago-shooting-domestic -violence_n_5bf576a6e4b0771fb6b4ceef.

2. Johnson R, Persad G, Sisti D. The Tarasoff rule: The implications of interstate variation and gaps in professional training. *J Am Acad Psychiatry Law*. 2014;42(4):469–477.

3. 45 CFR § 164.512(j). Uses and disclosures for which an authorization or opportunity to agree or object is not required. *Electronic Code of Federal Regulations.* https://www.ecfr.gov/current/title-45 /subtitle-A/subchapter-C/part-164/subpart-E/section-164.512.

4. Huecker MR, King KC, Jordan GA et al. *Domestic Violence.* StatPearls Publishing; 2023. https://www.ncbi.nlm.nih.gov/books /NBK499891/#.

5. Huecker et al. *Domestic Violence*; Abbott J, Johnson R, Koziol- McLain J, Lowenstein SR. Domestic violence against women. Incidence and prevalence in an emergency department population. *JAMA.* 1995 Jun 14;273(22): 1763–1767.

6. Table 2 in Rhodes KV, Kothari CL, Dichter M, Cerulli C, Wiley J, Marcus S. Intimate partner violence identification and response: time for a change in strategy. *J Gen Intern Med.* 2011 Aug;26(8):894–899.

7. Morral AR, Ramchand R, Smart R, et al. *The Science of Gun Policy: A Critical Synthesis of Research Evidence on the Effects of U.S. Gun Policies.* RAND Corporation; 2020.

8. American Academy of Pediatrics. Extreme risk protection orders (ERPO) or "red flag" laws. 2023. https://services.aap.org/en /advocacy/state-advocacy/extreme-risk-protection-orders-erpo-or -red-flag-laws/.

9. Grinshteyn E, Hemenway D. Violent death rates in the US compared to those of the other high-income countries. *Prev Med.* 2019;123(June):20–26.

10. Chicago doctor called 911 moments before ex-fiance killed her, 2 others. *CBS News.* November 21, 2018. https://www.cbsnews.com /news/chicago-hospital-shooting-dr-tamara-oneal-called-911 -moments-before-ex-fiance-juan-lopez-killed-her-2-others/.

11. Edwards B. A look at the troubled life of Mercy Hospital shooter Juan Lopez. *CBS Chicago.* November 20, 2018. https://chicago .cbslocal.com/2018/11/20/troubled-life-mercy-hospital-shooter -juan-lopez/; Rogers P. Autopsy results released for victims, gunman in Mercy Hospital shooting. *NBC 5 Chicago.* November 20, 2018. https://www.nbcchicago.com/news/local/autopsy

-results-released-for-victims-gunman-in-mercy-hospital-shooting
/168828/

12. Seidel J, Main F. Hospital shooter's history of threats no legal hurdle to owning gun. *Chicago Sun-Times.* November 20, 2018. https://chicago.suntimes.com/2018/11/20/18479467/hospital -shooter-s-history-of-threats-no-legal-hurdle-to-owning-gun.

13. Educational Fund to Stop Gun Violence. Extreme risk protection orders: An opportunity to save lives in Washington. September 2016. http://efsgv.org/wp-content/uploads/2016/09/FINAL -ERPO-complete-091916-1.pdf.

14. An Act Concerning Orders of Protection. Illinois Public Act 100–0607. Illinois General Assembly. https://www.ilga.gov /legislation/publicacts/fulltext.asp?Name=100-0607#:~:text =AN%20ACT%20concerning%20orders%20of%20protection .&text=Firearms%20Restraining%20Order%20Act.&text =person%20who%20shares%20a%20common%20dwelling%20 with%20the%20respondent.&text=receiving%20any%20firearms.

15. Centers for Disease Control and Prevention. Fast Facts: Preventing intimate partner violence. October 11, 2022., https://www.cdc.gov /violenceprevention/intimatepartnerviolence/fastfact.html.

16. Saltzman LE, Mercy JA, O'Carroll PW, et al. Weapon involvement and injury outcomes in family and intimate assaults. *JAMA.* 1992;267(22):3043–3047. doi:10.1001/jama.1992.034802200 61028.

17. Campbell JC, Webster D, Koziol-McLain J, et al. Risk factors for femicide in abusive relationships: results from a multisite case control study. *Am J Public Health.* 2003;93(7):1089–1097. doi:10.2105/ajph.93.7.1089.

18. Ackerman T. Methodist surgeon victim in apparent murder-suicide. *Houston Chronicle.* March 20, 2017. https://www.chron .com/neighborhood/fortbend/news/article/Methodist-surgeon -victim-in-apparent-11014770.php.

19. Federal Bureau of Investigation. Federal denials, Reasons Why the NICS Section Denies, November 30, 1998–October 31, 2018. https://www.fbi.gov/file-repository/federal_denials.pdf/view.

20. Morral AR, Ramchand R, Smart R, et al. *The Science of Gun Policy: A Critical Synthesis of Research Evidence on the Effects of U.S. Gun Policies.* RAND Corporation; 2020, 85–102, 111–119.

21. Campbell JC, Webster D, Koziol-McLain J, et al. Risk factors for femicide in abusive relationships: results from a multisite case control study. *Am J Public Health.* 2003 Jul;93(7):1089–1097.

14. Violence Interrupted

1. Wright L. Easy street. *Texas Monthly.* November 1982. https://www.texasmonthly.com/articles/easy-street/.

2. Church volunteer gunned down outside church on Houston's south side. *ABC13.* March 1, 2015. https://abc13.com/538307/.

3. Rich JA. *Wrong Place, Wrong Time.* Johns Hopkins University Press; 2019. p.57.

15. The Second Golden Hour of Trauma

1. CNN Hero Dr. Rob Gore. *CNN.* April 26, 2018. https://www.cnn.com/videos/us/2018/04/26/cnnheroes-gore-mixed.cnn.

2. O'Hare P. How Scotland stemmed the tide of knife crime. *BBC Scotland.* March 4, 2019. https://www.bbc.com/news/uk-scotland-45572691.

3. Operation ceasefire. Wikipedia. https://en.wikipedia.org/wiki/Operation_Ceasefire.

4. Toner K. Doctor works to save youth from violence before they reach his ER. *CNN.* December 9, 2018. https://www.cnn.com/2018/04/26/health/cnnheroes-rob-gore-kings-against-violence-initiative/index.html.

5. Grantham J. How the scene unfolded in Uvalde. ACEP *Now.* 2022;41(7):1, 6.

6. The White House. Fact sheet: More details on the Biden-Harris administration's investments in community violence interventions. April 7, 2021. https://www.whitehouse.gov/briefing-room/statements-releases/2021/04/07/fact-sheet-more-details-on-the-biden-harris-administrations-investments-in-community-violence-interventions/.

7. Prince George's Hospital Center, which opened in 1944, closed its doors to patients in 2021 and was replaced by Maryland Capital Region Medical Center. From 2007 to 2010, I worked there as an emergency medicine resident with the George Washington University emergency medicine program.

8. Brown DL. Prince George's neighborhoods make "Top 10 List of Richest Black Communities in America." *Washington Post*. January 23, 2015. https://www.washingtonpost.com/news/local /wp/2015/01/23/prince-georges-neighborhoods-make-top-10-list -of-richest-black-communities-in-america/.

9. DePillis L. Rich investors may have let Hahnemann Hospital go bankrupt. Now, they could profit from the land. *Philadelphia Tribune*. July 29, 2019. https://www.phillytrib.com/news/local _news/rich-investors-may-have-let-hahnemann-hospital-go -bankrupt-now-they-could-profit-from-the/article_283087b3 -13a4-533a-918d-3f1a1d869d59.html.

10. Delgado C. Making a difference: an interview with Sherman Spears. Colorlines. December 15, 1998. https://www.colorlines .com/articles/making-difference-interview-sherman-spears.

11. Smith R, Dobbins S, Evans A, et al. Hospital-based violence intervention: risk reduction resources that are essential for success. *J Trauma Acute Care Surg*. 2013;74(4):976–980.

12. Cheng TL, Haynie D, Brenner R, et al. Effectiveness of a mentor-implemented, violence prevention intervention for assault-injured youths presenting to the emergency department: results of a randomized trial. *Pediatrics*. 2008;122(5):938–946.

13. Cooper C, Eslinger DM, Stolley PD. Hospital-based violence intervention programs work. *J Trauma*. 2006;61(3):534–540.

14. Zun LS, Downey L, Rosen J. The effectiveness of an ED-based violence prevention program. *Am J Emerg Med*. 2006;24(1):8–13.

15. Emmy Betz. Twitter post. November 11, 2018. 9:28 A.M. https:// twitter.com/EmmyBetz/status/1061641728615112704?s=20.

16. We Don't Have to Wait to Act

1. The perpetrator of the Las Vegas shooting also killed himself. However, I chose not to include the names of killers in the manuscript of this book and, in this case, in the enumeration of the dead. After the shooting, two additional victims (Kimberly Gervais and Samanta Arjune) died as a consequence of their injuries sustained that day. The names of some killers may appear in the titles of citations used to source this book.

2. Dark C, Sakran J, Fischer K. History has its eye on us: Clinicians should rally behind "This Is Our Lane." *Health Affairs*. February 21, 2019. DOI:10.1377/hblog20190221.8649.

3. Morral AR, Ramchand R, Smart R, et al. *The Science of Gun Policy: A Critical Synthesis of Research Evidence on the Effects of U.S. Gun Policies*. RAND Corporation; 2020.

4. Alexander Hamilton did not want to duel with Aaron Burr but felt it was necessary to maintain his honor and reputation if he wanted to retain the ability to influence public policy in the future. He wrote: "The ability to be in future useful, whether in resisting mischief or effecting good, in those crises of public affairs, which seem likely to happen, would probably be inseparable from a conformity with public prejudice in this particular." These are the last words Hamilton wrote with regard to his impending duel with Burr. Hamilton A. Statement on impending duel with Aaron Burr, [28 June–10 July 1804]. National Archives. https://founders.archives .gov/documents/Hamilton/01-26-02-0001-0241.

5. Morral et al. *The Science of Gun Policy*, xxvi.

6. Concealed carry. Giffords Law Center. https://giffords.org/lawcenter /gun-laws/policy-areas/guns-in-public/concealed-carry/.

7. Gounder C. How do criminals get their guns? Interview with Lonny Pulkrabek, Daniel Webster, Cassandra Crifasi, and Harold Pollack. *American Diagnosis: Gun Violence in America*. Podcast. May 16, 2019. https://podcasts.apple.com/us/podcast/american -diagnosis-with-dr-celine-gounder/id1282044849?i=1000438 237343.

8. Donohue JJ, Aneja A, Weber K. Right-to-carry laws and violent crime: a comprehensive assessment using panel data and a state-level synthetic control analysis (June 2019). *Journal of Empirical Legal Studies*. 2019;16(2):198–247. https://doi.org/10.1111/jels.12219.

Epilogue

1. Rees CA, Monuteaux MC, Steidley I, et al. Trends and disparities in firearm fatalities in the United States, 1990–2021. *JAMA Netw Open*. 2022;5(11):e2244221.

2. Stark DE, Shah NH. Funding and publication of research on gun violence and other leading causes of death. *JAMA*. 2017;317(1):84–85.

INDEX

Page numbers in italics refer to figures and tables.

140; homicides involving firearms and, 136, 138; lack of safe places, 134–35; murder-suicides, 58; restraining orders and, 136, 140, 172, 175; Tarasoff doctrine and, 133–34
Duncan, Carmelo, 12
duty to retreat, 70, 176–77

emergency medicine, 18, 49, 135
Emory Center for Injury Control at Rollins School of Public Health, 31
epidemiologists, 19, 20, 22, 97

family fire, 99, 126
FBI (Federal Bureau of Investigation), 100, 103, 104. *See also* NICS (National Instant Criminal Background Check System)
Federal Firearms Act (1938), 38
felony convictions, *98*, 100
fingerprinting, as vetting for firearm permits, 80
firearm/gun safety, 82, 98, 113; NRA course on, 112, 116; physicians' role in, 115; storage of firearms and ammunition, 124–25
firearms/guns, 3, 20; accidental deaths and, 126; constitutional right to bear arms, 24; criminals' acquisition of, 102; for hunting, 10, 68, 90; intimate partner violence and, 47; as keepsakes, 68; licensing for, 38; mosquitoes as disease vectors compared to, 19–20; physicians as gun owners, 1, 20, 64, 67–69; regulation and restrictions on, 38; restricted availability of, 41; for self-protection, 10, 30, 36, 68, 73; shotguns, 68, 72, 73, 78–79; for sports (clay and range shooting), 10, 68, 90; statistics on deaths and injuries from, 24, 61, 90, 169, 181, 183; toy guns as danger for Black children, 70; as vectors for violence, 74, 97, 158, 181. *See also* assault weapons; handguns

firearms purchases, 81, 101, 172; categories of people denied purchases of, 87, 100; federal licensed dealers, 100, 102, 103, 107, 123; Gun Control Act (1968) and, 100; licenses and permits for, 172, 174; minimum age for, 122–24, *123*, 174; person-to-person, 87, 101
Fischer, Dr. Kyle, 60, 104, 141, 163–65, 167, 170; at Gun Safety Forum (Las Vegas, 2020), 171; as HAVI policy director, 59
Fix NICS Act (2017), 104, 106
Fleegler, Dr. Eric, 121
Ford, Gerald, 81
Frederick, Karl, 38

Gaye, Marvin, shooting death of, 27–29, 30, 36
Gervais, Kimberly, 204n1
Giffords Courage, 171
Giffords Law Center to Prevent Gun Violence, 101
Gingrich, Newt, 44
Giordano, Dr. Joseph, 85–86
Goldfrank, Dr. Lewis R., 19
Gordon-Burroughs, Dr. Sherilyn, 139
Gordy, Dr. Stephanie, 71–74, 79, 140, 144
Gore, Dr. Rob, 158, 160–61, 162, 165
"gun buddy" idea, 117, 119, 120
gun control, 56, 81, 89, 168
Gun Control Act (1968), 100
gun lobby. *See* NRA (National Rifle Association)
Gun Safety Forum (Las Vegas, 2020), 171
gun shop owners, 119, 120
gunshot victims, 21, 34, 163–65; in author's family, 6–7, 8, 9, 11; author's friend Lee shot by brother, 145–56, 166; history of medical literature on, 39–40, 187n4; killed in their homes, 32, 36; nonfatal wounds, 61; numbers of, 1, 9, 10

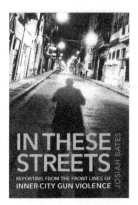
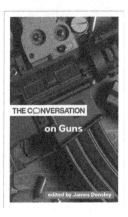
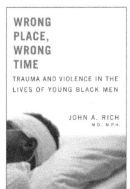